West China Hospital, West China S⬚

West China Series of Auxiliary Textbook of Diagnostics

Graphics-Sequenced Interpretation of ECG

心电图图形顺序解读（英文版）

Author Rui Zeng

编　著　曾　锐

Reviser Zhi Zeng

审　校　曾　智

人民卫生出版社

PEOPLE'S MEDICAL PUBLISHING HOUSE

图书在版编目（CIP）数据

心电图图形顺序解读 =Graphics-sequenced interpretation of
ECG：英文 / 曾锐编著 .—北京：人民卫生出版社，2015
　　ISBN 978-7-117-20219-0

　　Ⅰ. ①心… 　Ⅱ. ①曾… 　Ⅲ. ①心电图 – 医学院校 – 教材 –
英文 　Ⅳ. ①R540.4

　　中国版本图书馆 CIP 数据核字（2015）第 014066 号

人卫社官网　**www.pmph.com**	出版物查询，在线购书	
人卫医学网　**www.ipmph.com**	医学考试辅导，医学数	
	据库服务，医学教育	
	资源，大众健康资讯	

Graphics-Sequenced Interpretation of ECG
心电图图形顺序解读（英文版）

编　　著：曾　锐
出版发行：人民卫生出版社（中继线 010-59780011）
地　　址：北京市朝阳区潘家园南里 19 号
邮　　编：100021
E - mail：pmph @ pmph.com
购书热线：010-59787592　010-59787584　010-65264830
印　　刷：北京汇林印务有限公司
经　　销：新华书店
开　　本：850×1168　1/32　　印张：6.5
字　　数：175 千字
版　　次：2015 年 3 月第 1 版　2015 年 3 月第 1 版第 1 次印刷
标准书号：ISBN 978-7-117-20219-0/R · 20220
定　　价：25.00 元

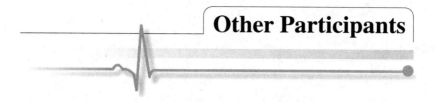

Other Participants

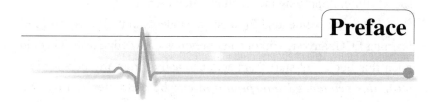

Preface

Diagnostics is an important area of medical knowledge and the interpretation of electrocardiogram (ECG) is an indispensable component of diagnostics. As a basic medical test in clinical settings, ECG plays a significant role in the diagnosis of cardiovascular diseases and is being used more frequently than before, since the incidence of cardiovascular diseases has been noticeably increased.

Due to the abstract nature of the basic theoretical knowledge of ECG, its scattered characteristics, and tedious and difficult-to-remember subject matter, it is difficult for teachers to teach and for students to learn. As a result, some students tend to be unenthusiastic about learning about ECG, some resist learning it, and others give it up altogether. If these problems are left unsolved, ECG teaching may fail to meet its teaching requirements, and subsequently affect the ability of medical students to correctly read ECGs in their future clinical work. Therefore, we must change traditional teaching ideas and optimize teaching methods to improve the quality of ECG teaching.

In order to make medical students to master the fundamental knowledge and skills of ECG reading and interpretation in a limited time, our young doctor Rui Zeng summarized his understanding of ECG based on his experience in clinical teaching and combined it with the contents in the traditional ECG outline. Altogether this resulted in a new approach in ECG teaching——*Graphics-sequenced interpretation*. By implementing this new approach, he has been successful in improving the teaching effectiveness.

This book is intended for medical students in their early stage of learning ECG; anyone without any previous knowledge of ECG could open this book and start from scratch easily. From my perspective, *Graphics-sequenced interpretation* can be characterized by two keywords. The first one is graphics. It means that when teaching ECG, schematic diagrams of normal and abnormal ECGs are shown to students. This intuitive approach could make morphology of normal and abnormal ECG clearly understood. The second keyword is sequence. It means that when students learn to analyze ECG, they should follow the specific sequence of ECG waveform generation, namely, the analysis of heart rate and rhythm, the P wave, P-R interval period, QRS wave, ST segment and T wave, Q-T interphase, and U wave. After getting used to this simple and practical method in ECG interpretation, students will discover how easy it is to read an ECG strip and at the same time avoid omissions in the diagnosis of abnormal conditions.

As a supplementary reading in the West China Diagnostics series, I sincerely anticipate the publication of this book. It will open the door to ECG learning for all medical students as well as clinicians working in primary settings and be of great use in their daily work or study.

West China School of Medicine
West China Hospital
Sichuan University

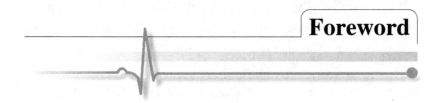

Foreword

I first came in close contact with the electrocardiogram when I was a third year medical student in 2001. More than 10 years have passed but I could remember it clearly as if it happened yesterday. I was not a diligent student back then and was reluctant to learn anything that requires careful contemplation and full attention in class. Therefore for me, ECG was merely questions I had to answer on a test and failed to preoccupy any territory of neither my mind nor my heart. For all that I am concerned, I could discriminate an ECG from an X-ray image, CT or MRI scan when I see it.

In 2005, as a second year graduate student, I began my clinical rotation which lasted for more than two years. Cardiology was the first specialty I came across. Fear and pressure with an intensity exceeding any past experiences overtook me during my early days in the department. The main reason for that is my incapacity to deal with different types of cardiac arrhythmia. My graduate study was not focused on cardiology (rather gastroenterology) and neither did I engage in clinical rotation or systemic study of the ECG in my years as an undergraduate. Confronted with sudden onsets of supraventricular tachycardia and ventricular tachycardia, all I knew was that the patient's heart beat was very fast and nothing else. Frantic and distressed, I could only constantly turn to the chief resident for help (the chief resident back then was Mr. Qing YANG who is quite well known as a blogger now). Every time I saw him taking the ECG from my hands calmly and explain his analysis to me, I would be filled with respect and admiration, and could not stop asking myself, why one piece ECG could embody so many interesting interpretations. From that point on, I felt ECG is no longer a question on a test but a common clinical procedure that demands to be learnt well. However, I never came around to studying it because of the overwhelming load of clinical work.

In 2007, the hospital I worked at set the requirement that all PhD students with a specialty (I transferred to cardiology during my PhD study) have to work for three months as associate chief resident. For me it was another three months filled with panic. In our department the main responsibility of the associate chief resident was to assist the chief resident in ward management, and deal with emergencies when he or she is attending clinical consultations. Days felt like years to me back then because I am no longer an ordinary resident but someone all the other residents turn to when confronted with difficult problems. Those memories still scare me to this moment. Fortunately, nothing disastrous happened and I made it safe through those three months.

A year later, funded by the China Scholarship Council, I was able to go to the Faculty of Medicine of Monash University in Australia on a joint PhD program. My stay in Australia lasted for more than three years, a lot longer than I had originally planned. It wasn't until 2012 after I had finished my post doctoral research that I returned to work at the West China Hospital.

During my stay abroad, I carefully read through many books about ECG, most of which were borrowed from the library of Monash Medical Center. The ones that inspired me the most was *The Clinical Analysis and Diagnosis of ECG* by Dr. Xinmin Zhang, *Rapid ECG Interpretation* by Dr. M. Gabriel Khan and *The ECG Made Easy* series by Dr. John R. Hampton, which laid the theoretical foundation for forming my own understanding of ECG recognition.

When I returned, I started my job as chief resident under the guidance of my medical group director. Every month, the interns, graduate students or residents in my group would switch and we are met with new faces. The future doctors who are on their rotation loved listening to my interpretation of ECG. Month after month, I would repeat the same explanation and re-draw the same ECG strip. Eventually, an idea sprang up in my head that I could explain the parts that are difficult to understand and write the rest down for others to read in a book, which is not only more efficient but greatly reduces my work load.

With this thought, the *Graphics-sequenced interpretation of ECG* gradually came into being. It is a collection of my understanding of ECG, hoping to help readers study ECG from an easy and practical perspective.

The date I finished writing is coincidentally the first birthday of my son, to whom I dedicate this book. I would also like to thank my lovely wife, who sacrificed much for our family, for her consideration and understanding. Both of you are the treasure of my life.

In view of my limited scope and depth, there are inevitably places of error or omission which all readers are welcome to rectify, for the improvement of the book in later editions.

Rui Zeng

Department of Cardiology, West China Hospital,
Sichuan University
June 21st, 2014

Contents

Chapter 1

Basic Knowledge of ECG

Section 1   The First Sight of ECG

This is a normal standard 12-lead ECG (Figure 1-1). What can you see when you get a first sight of this ECG?

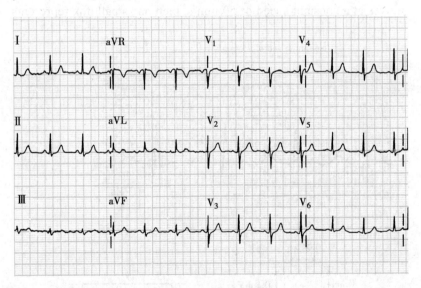

Figure 1-1   Normal ECG.

First, you will find that there are a lot of square boxes. Second, you will find that there are many confusing waves. Finally, you may also find that there are some Roman numerals (I , II , III) as well as some combinations of letters and numbers (aVR, aVL, aVF, V_1, V_2, V_3, V_4, V_5, V_6).

Therefore, in order to fully appreciate the world of ECG, we first need to accomplish some preparation, in other words, to get familiar with the electrocardiogram. Let's start with the boxes.

I. What's the Connotation of the Boxes?

All the boxes are squares with 1 mm on a side. The horizontal line of the boxes (horizontal ordinate) represents time. The length of time each box can vary, depending on the constant speed of the graph paper. Normally when the graph paper moves at a constant speed of 25 mm/s, one box represents 0.04 s (40 ms); when the graph paper moves at a constant speed of 50 mm/s, then one small box represents

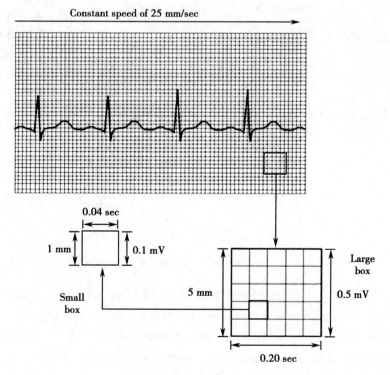

Figure 1-2   25 mm/s paper speed.

0.02 s (20 ms), and the rest can be done in the same fashion. The vertical line of the box (vertical ordinate), otherwise, represents voltage, 0.1 mV per small box normally (Figure 1-2).

Every 25 boxes (5×5) contribute to a large box, so the large box is also a square each of which represents 0.2 s (200 ms) on the horizontal ordinate and 0.5 mV on the vertical ordinate (Figure 1-2).

II. What Are the Confusing Waves?

After boxes, we came to see the *confusing* waves. Before we explain the waves, we should review some basic cardiac electrophysiology.

The electrical impulses is derived from a special pace-making area in the right atrium called sinoatrial (SA) node and then triggers the contraction of heart in course of its gradual conduction. Figure 1-3 shows the whole process of how the impulse is produced by the SA node and spread to the entire heart. The impulse would first move

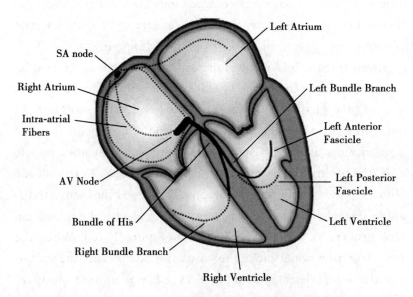

Figure 1-3   Cardiac electrical conduction.

through right and left atrium, then reach the atrioventricular (AV) node through the conduction of internodal pathways. After the impulse having reached the AV node, the depolarization would be delayed for a while. Finally the impulse moves to stimulate the ventricular muscle through the bundles of His and the left and right bundle branches. It's noteworthy that the SA node and ventricular muscle have no stable resting potential and the SA node has automaticity, meaning it possess the feature of automatic depolarization and repolarization thus acting as the pacemaker of the heart. Normally, the cardiac muscles, conduction system aside, are unable to depolarize automatically, they can only be stimulated by the impulse from the other part of the heart.

The Depolarization and Repolarization of the Heart

When at resting state, for a cardiac muscle cell specifically, the positively charged ions are located at the outer side of the cell membrane and the negatively charged ions are located at the inner side of the cell membrane, therefore, rendering the cell at a state of equilibrium described as *positive outside and negative inside* or polarized (Figure 1-4A). When the cell membrane is stimulated by the outer electric activity, the negatively charged ions move outward whereas the positively charged ions move inward, to alter the state to negative outside and positive inside. This process is called depolarization (Figure 1-4B). At the recovery phase of cardiac muscle cells, the positively charged ions, again, move back to the outside of the cell membrane, and the negatively charged ions move to the inside. Thereby the cell returns to a state of electrical equilibrium. This process is called repolarization (Figure 1-4C). When the depolarization wave moves towards the electrodes, the galvo-recorder would detect and record a wave that is upward (positive) (Figure 1-5A). When the depolarization wave moves away from the

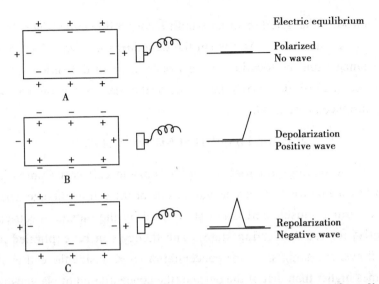

Figure 1-4　Polarization, depolarization and repolarization of cardiac muscle cell.

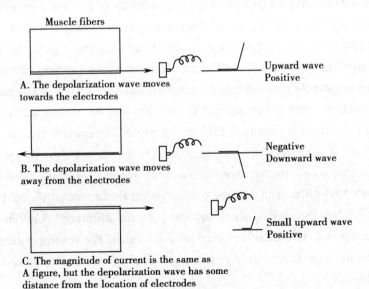

Figure 1-5　Relationship between current flow direction and ECG wave pattern.

electrodes, the galvo-recorder would record a downward (negative) wave (Figure 1-5B). And when the depolarization wave has some distance from the location of electrodes, a small deflection would be recorded (Figure 1-5C), that's one of the reasons for low voltage occurrence in the ECG.

Resting Potential of Myocardial Cell

The resting potential of cardiac muscle cell is the potential difference between the inside and outside of the cell membrane when the cardiac muscle cell is not stimulated by the outside electrical activities (at the resting state). The theory can be explained as follows: at resting state, the concentration of K^+ inside the cell is 30 times higher than that of the outside (the concentration of Na^+ outside the cell is 30 times higher than that of the inside). In addition, the cell membrane has a relatively high permeability to K^+, and a relatively low permeability to Na^+ and organic negatively charged ions A^-. As a result, K^+ can diffuse from inside of the membrane to the outside under the concentration difference (concentration gradient) whereas the negatively charged ions A^- cannot diffuse with K^+ in the opposite direction. With the process of K^+ moving out, the membrane would slowly form a potential difference which is *negative inside and positive outside*. Such potential difference would slow down the process of K^+ further moving out, until reaching a point when the potential difference and the concentration difference of K^+ balance out. Then the moving stops and this potential difference between the inside and outside of the membrane is called the resting potential (Figure 1-6). Normally, the resting potential of cardiac muscle cells is −90 mV.

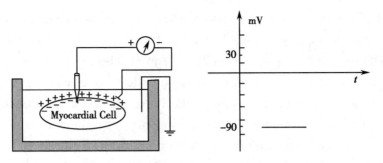

Figure 1-6　Resting potential of cardiac muscle cells.

Action potential of Cardiac Muscle Cells

If the cell is stimulated properly on the basis of resting potential, a rapid and transient fluctuation of the membrane potential will be triggered. Such fluctuation in the membrane is called action potential. Action potential is the sign of cardiac excitation.

According to the change of potential, action potential of cardiac muscle cell can be divided into five phases (Figure 1-7) as phase 0, phase 1, phase 2, phase 3 and phase 4. Its mechanism is as follows. When the cardiac cell receives a certain level of stimulus, the stimulus would trigger the opening of Na^+ channel in the cell membrane and increase of Na^+ inflow. Under the dual effect of both the electric

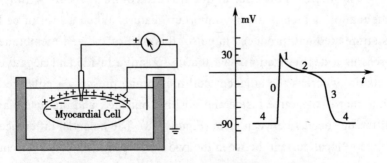

Figure 1-7　Action potential of cardiac muscle cells.

gradient and the concentration gradient, Na^+ move inside the cell membrane rapidly and result in a rapid increase of potential inside which is higher than the outside (+30 mV). The cell membrane is then at a positive inside and negative outside depolarized state. This process is the 0 phase of action potential. Na^+ channel is fast channel, activation and inactivation both happen in very short time, and when the cell depolarization reaches a peak, the potential inside will decline with the closing and inactivation of Na^+ channel, that is, the repolarization process of cardiac muscle. The repolarization process is rather slow, including phase 1, phase 2, and phase 3. At phase 1, the cause for action potential waveform is the outflow of K^+. The waveform at phase 2 is relatively flattened so it is called the *plateau phase* or the *slow recovery state*, the mechanism of this plateau is mainly the relatively balanced state of outflow (K^+) and inflow (Ca^{2+}) of ions. The action waveform of phase 3 is rather steep. With the inactivation of Ca^+ channel and massive opening of K^+ channel, the process of repolarization is accelerated apparently (the rapid recovery phase), and eventually recover to the previous negative inside and positive outside state, otherwise, to the resting state.

Conduction of Action Potential

The action potential could travel around the cell without attenuation, which is a very important feature. When a spot of cell is stimulated and produces impulse, this part of the cell membrane presents a depolarization state that is 'positive inside and negative outside' whereas the adjacent cell membrane presents a polarized state that is 'negative inside and positive outside', and the potential difference occurs between them (Figure 1-8). The potential difference renders 'local current' between the two parts. When the local current begins to move, it results in the elevation of membrane potential in

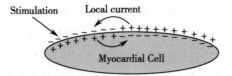

Figure 1-8　Conduction of action potentials.

the adjacent cell membrane (the potential difference between the inside and outside of the membrane deceases). When the membrane potential reaches the threshold potential, it will excite the adjacent part to form action potential. In such case, one part of excitation in the membrane can travel through the whole cell membrane by the local current, producing new action potential successively until the whole cardiac cell is excited.

Relationships of Depolarization, Repolarization and Waveforms on ECG

The recording of action potential is actually the recording of inner cell potential changes during the process of depolarization and repolarization in one single cell (Figure 1-9A). What is recorded in

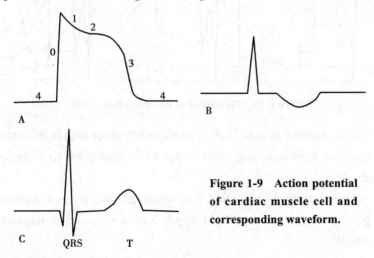

Figure 1-9　Action potential of cardiac muscle cell and corresponding waveform.

the Figure 1-9B is the outer cell potential changes of one single cell during the process of depolarization and repolarization. The waveform of ECG is the potential changes of the whole heart (all cardiac muscle cells) during the process of depolarization and repolarization.

III. The Meaning of Roman Numerals and Combinations of Letters and Mumerals

The Conventional 12 Leads

The Roman numerals (I , II & III) in ECG, and several combinations of letters and numerals (aVR, aVL, aVF, V_1, V_2, V_3, V_4, V_5, V_6) represent the leads on ECG. It consists of three standard leads (I , II & III), three augmented leads (aVR, aVL, aVF) and six chest leads (V_1, V_2, V_3, V_4, V_5, V_6).

Standard leads, or bipolar limb leads (Figure 1-10):

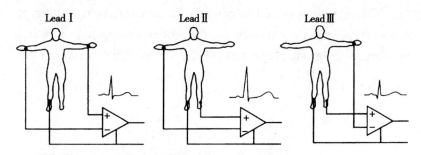

Figure 1-10　Placement of standard limb leads.

First standard lead, or lead I , in which left upper limb is connected to positive electrode and right upper limb connected to negative electrode.

Second standard lead, or lead II, in which left lower limb is connected to positive electrode and right upper limb connected to negative electrode.

Third standard lead, or lead Ⅲ, in which left lower limb is connected to positive electrode and left upper limb connected to negative electrode.

Augmented unipolar limb leads (Figure 1-11):

Augmented right upper limb lead, or lead aVR, in which the

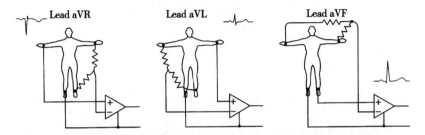

Figure1-11   Placement of augmented unipolar limb leads.

electrode is placed on right upper limb.

Augmented left upper limb lead, or lead aVL, in which the electrode is placed on left upper limb.

Augmented left lower limb lead, or lead aVF, in which the electrode is placed on left lower limb.

Chest leads: otherwise ,V leads are unipolar. (Figure 1-12):

Lead V_1: the electrode is placed in the fourth intercostal space to the right of the sternum.

Lead V_2: the electrode is placed in the fourth intercostal space to

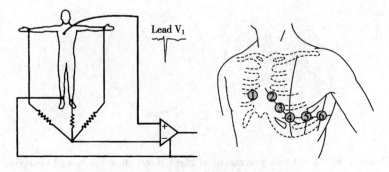

Figure 1-12   Placement of chest leads.

the left of the sternum.

Lead V_3: the electrode is placed in the midpoint between V_2 and V_4.

Lead V_4: the electrode is placed in the fifth intercostal space in the midclavicular line.

Lead V_5: the electrode is placed at the intersection of left anterior axillary line and V_4 electrode level.

Lead V_6: the electrode is placed at the intersection of left midaxillary line and V_4 electrode level.

Other Special Leads

Right-sided chest leads (Figure 1-13A):

Chest leads V_1 to V_6 are placed at the same position on the right chest, and thus labeled as V_{1R} to V_{6R}. Right-sided chest leads are mainly used to make clinical diagnosis of right ventricular hypertrophy, dextrocardia and right ventricular infarction.

Posterior-wall leads (Figure 1-13B):

Electrodes that are placed at intersections of V_4 level and posterior axillary line, left scapular line and to the left of spinal

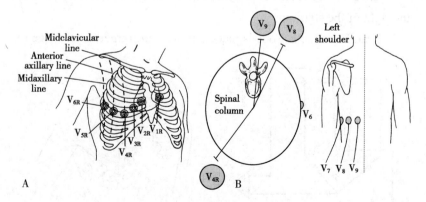

Figure 1-13　Electrode placement of right-sided chest leads and posterior-wall leads.

column are labeled posterior-wall lead V_7, V_8 and V_9 respectively.

An 18-Lead ECG:

In certain clinical context, an 18-lead ECG will be adopted, including three right-sided chest leads (V_{3R}, V_{4R} & $V_{5R)}$ and three posterior-wall leads (V_7, V_8 & V_9) besides the conventional 12 leads.

The Lead Axis

The lead axis of a certain lead is defined as an imaginary line extending from negative electrode to positive electrode of the lead. Usually, an arrowhead is used to represent the positive electrode. Axes are mainly categorized as limb leads (Figure 1-14) and chest leads (Figure 1-14). For example, in lead I, the positive electrode is placed on left upper limb and the negative electrode on right upper limb. Therefore, the axis for lead I starts from right upper limb to left upper limb (from negative to positive), and the direction is shown in Figure 1-14. In lead II, positive electrode is placed on left lower limb and negative electrode on right upper limb. Therefore, the axis for lead II starts from right upper limb to left lower limb (from negative to positive), and the direction is shown in Figure 1-14. Following the method discussed above, you could work out directions of the rest of axes by yourself.

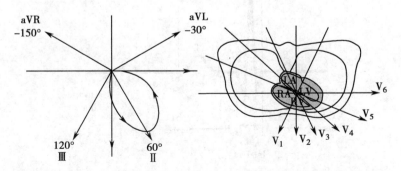

Figure 1-14   Hexaxial reference system and cardiac axes in horizontal plane.

Axes for limb leads are in cardiac frontal plane, indicating distribution of vectors in the frontal plane and is called **hexaxial reference system.** Axes of chest leads are in cardiac horizontal plane, indicating distribution of vectors in the horizontal plane.

Section 2   Configuration and Representation of Waves & Segments in ECG

Electrical impulse discharged from sinoatrial node activates atria and ventricle and sequentially causes depolarization and repolarization, producing a series of potential differences on the body surface, which are recorded as ECG (Figure 1-15). Waves in ECG are labeled as P, Q, R, S, T and U, all of which were defined during early ECG development. Among all the waves, P, T and U wave are single deflection, while Q, R and S waves are grouped together to form QRS complex.

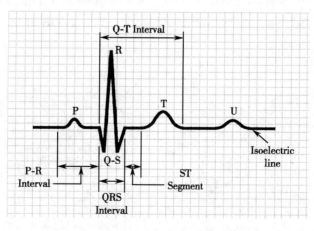

Figure 1-15   Waves and segments in ECG.

P Wave

P wave is the first deflection in a group of waves. It represents left and right atrial depolarization. P wave is upright (including rounded, notched, double-peaked, tall-peaked), or may have biphasic and inverted morphology (Figure 1-16).

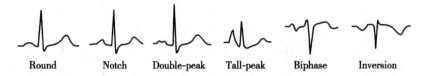

| Round | Notch | Double-peak | Tall-peak | Biphase | Inversion |

Figure 1-16   Common configuration of P wave.

P-R Interval

P-R interval refers to the interval from the beginning of P wave to the beginning of QRS complex, and measures the time during which depolarization begins in atria and travels through internodal pathways, atrioventricular junction, bundle of His, left and right bundle branch and their fascicles and Purkinje fibers to depolarize ventricles.

QRS Complex

QRS complex is a group of deflections that has greater amplitude and consists of Q, R and S waves. It represents depolarization in left and right ventricles. A typical QRS complex includes three consecutive deflections. The first negative deflection is called Q wave, the first (also post-Q wave) positive deflection is called R wave, and the negative deflection after R wave is called S wave, altogether comprise the QRS complex.

Occasionally, a positive deflection follows S wave and thus is called R′ wave (R-prime). If R′ wave occurs, then a negative deflection follows, and it's called S' wave. If its amplitude is less than 0.5 mV, then the wave is represented by a lowercase letter q, r or s. If its amplitude is greater than or equal to 0.5 mV, then the wave is represented by a capital letter Q, R or S. Common configurations of the QRS complex are in Figure 1-17.

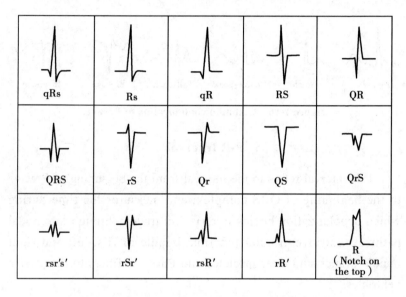

Figure 1-17   Common configurations of the QRS complex.

ST Segment

ST segment is the line that connects the end of QRS complex and the beginning of T wave, representing the slow process of ventricular depolarization. See Figure 1-18 for the common variants of ST segment.

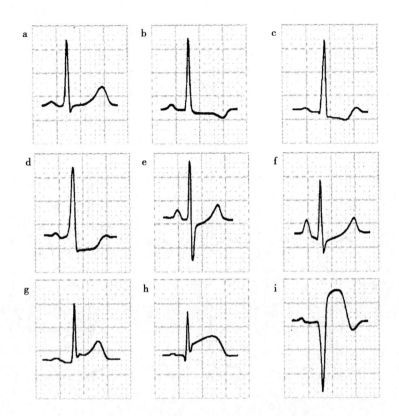

Figure 1-18   Common deviations of ST segment.
a: normal ST segment *b*: horizontal ST depression *c*: down-sloping ST depression *d*: horizontal ST depression *e*: J point depression *f*: up-sloping ST depression *g*: concave ST elevation *h*: convex ST elevation *i*: convex ST elevation

T Wave

T wave is a deflection that follows ST segment and represents rapid repolarization across the ventricle. Like P wave, the T wave has multiple variants: upright, notched, flattening, positive-negative biphasic, negative-positive biphasic and inverted. See Figure 1-19.

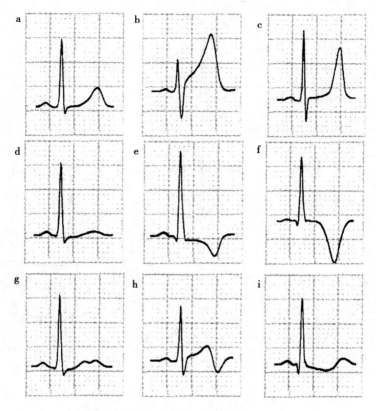

Figure 1-19 Common deviations of T wave.

a: normal T wave *b*: peaked T wave *c*: tall peaked T wave *d*: flattening T wave
e: asymmetrically inverted T wave *f*: symmetrically inverted T wave *g*: 'camel
hump' T wave *h*: positive-negative biphasic T wave *i*: negative-positive biphasic
T wave

Q-T Interval

Q-T interval measures the time from the beginning of QRS
complex to the end of T wave, representing the whole process
of ventricular depolarization and repolarization. Q-T interval is
frequently affected by heart rate. When heart rate is between 60

and 100 bpm, duration of Q-T interval is 0.32 to 0.44 seconds. To eliminate its effect on Q-T interval, we can calculate a corrected value of Q-T interval (Q-Tc) by the following equation: Q-Tc=Q-T/√RR, which represents the Q-T interval at 60 bpm.

U Wave

U wave is a small deflection that follows T wave, and its generating mechanism remains unknown. More details will be discussed in Chapter 7.

Section 3   Graphics-Sequenced Interpretation of ECG

After learning the basics of ECG in previous sections, now we come to the part learning how to interpret ECG. Based on experience of years of clinical teaching, the author had summarized a simple and practical study method—**Graphics-Sequenced Interpretation of ECG**. There are two key words here, one is ECG Graphics, which means understanding the mechanisms that cause normal and abnormal ECG tracing and memorizing them based on Graphics. The other one is **sequence**, which means interpreting an ECG tracing following the order that it is generated (P wave, P-R interval, QRS complex, ST segment, T wave, Q-T interval, U wave). In this way, analysis of ECG can be quite easy and would not miss any significant diagnostic information. In following chapters, we will discuss how to use this method to interpret ECG. In general, when you come across an ECG tracing, you should follow these steps:

- **Step 1: Is the rhythm regular? Estimate heart rate based on the rhythm.**
- **Step 2: Analyze P wave**

- **Step 3: Analyze P-R interval**
- **Step 4: Analyze QRS complex**
- **Step 5: Analyze ST segment**
- **Step 6: Analyze T wave**
- **Step 7: Other ECG variants**

Section 4 Calculating Heart Rate in Regular or Irregular Rhythm

Regular Rhythm

When the rhythm is regular in an ECG tracing, heart rate is determined by two successive P-R intervals. In previous sections, we have studied the significance and function of boxes, now let us review this part. In every horizontal axis, a small box represents time, which stands for 40 ms; 5 small boxes comprise a large box, which stands for 200 ms; 5 large boxes grouped together count exactly 1 second (Figure 1-20).

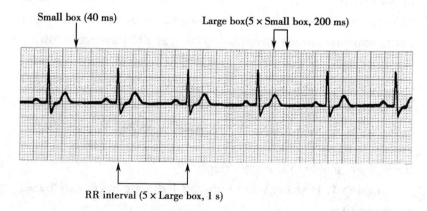

Small box (40 ms)

Large box(5 × Small box, 200 ms)

RR interval (5 × Large box, 1 s)

Figure 1-20   Useful data.

Therefore, based on the understanding of boxes, when the rhythm is regular we can calculate heart rate by counting the boxes. See Figure 1-21 for more details.

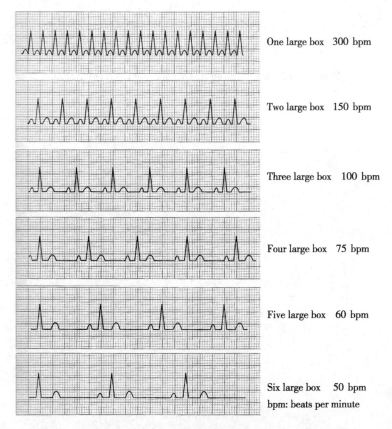

One large box 300 bpm

Two large box 150 bpm

Three large box 100 bpm

Four large box 75 bpm

Five large box 60 bpm

Six large box 50 bpm

bpm: beats per minute

Figure 1-21 Heart rate and corresponding boxes in regular rhythm.

Irregular Rhythm

If the rhythm were irregular in an ECG tracing, we could firstly count heart beats in 6 seconds, and then multiply the count by 10 to get heart rate. For example, in Figure 1-22, the count of heart beat in

6 seconds is 10, and then the heart rate is: 10×10=100 bpm.

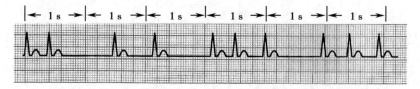

Figure 1-22   Calculating heart rate in irregular rhythm.

Chapter 2

P Wave

The P wave is the first wavelet in the P-QRS-T complex, representing the potential changes produced by the depolarization of the left and right atria.

Section 1   Sinus P Wave

Normal sinus P wave generate from the sinus node, which is located at the junction of the superior vena cava and the right atrium. The sinus node discharges electrical impulses to activate the atria, forming a depolarization vector in atria, which mainly points to lower left (Figure 2-1). Considering the hexaxial reference system and the axes of chest leads, we can see that the atrial depolarization vectors are positive in leads I, II, aVF, V_4 to V_6, following the pattern in

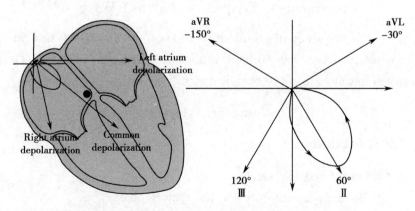

Figure 2-1   Cause of the morphology of sinus P wave.

lead II; while they are negative in lead aVR, obviously opposite to the pattern in lead II. Then we can draw a brief conclusion about the ECG features of the normal sinus P wave.

[Characteristics of electrocardiogram of the normal sinus P wave]

1. P wave in sinus rhythm appears small, rounded, and upright in leads I, II, aVF, V_4 to V_6.

2. Sinus P wave is inverted in lead aVR.

3. In other leads it can be upright, inverted, or biphasic (half upright, half inverted).

4. Normal duration of sinus P wave should be less than 0.12 s, and amplitude of P wave less than 0.25 mV in limb leads or amplitude less than 0.2 mV in chest leads.

[ECG Tracing] P wave is upright in lead II, and inverted in lead aVR (Figure 2-2).

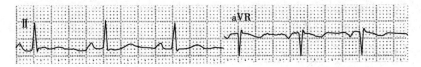

Figure 2-2   Sinus P wave.

I. Abnormality in Frequency of Sinus P Wave

The frequency of normal P wave is 60 to 100 bpm. When the frequency is less than 60 bpm, it is sinus bradycardia (Figure 2-3); when it is more than 100 bpm, it is sinus tachycardia (Figure 2-4).

Sinus Bradycardia

[ECG Recognition]

1. Sinus P wave is present.
2. The frequency of P wave is less than 60 bpm.
3. It may be accompanied by sinus arrhythmia.

[ECG Tracing] (Figure 2-3)

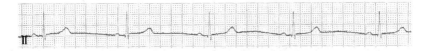

Figure 2-3　Sinus bradycardia.

Sinus Tachycardia

[ECG Recognition]

> 1. Sinus rhythm.
> 2. The frequency of P wave is more than 100 bpm and maybe higher in children.

[ECG Tracing] (Figure 2-4)

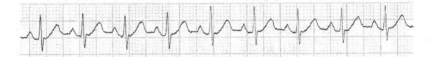

Figure 2-4　Sinus tachycardia.

II. Abnormality in Voltage or Duration of Sinus P Wave (Atrial Enlargement)

Since the sinus node is located at the junction of the superior vena cava and the right atrium, the electrical impulses discharged by the excited sinus node first activate the right atrium, then the left atrium. The depolarization of all atria is reflected by P wave on ECG, therefore the right atrial depolarization takes the first 2/3 of P wave and the depolarization of the left atrium takes the last 2/3, which means the middle 1/3 of the P wave is the sum of synchronal depolarization of right and left atria (Figure 2-5). Normal P wave

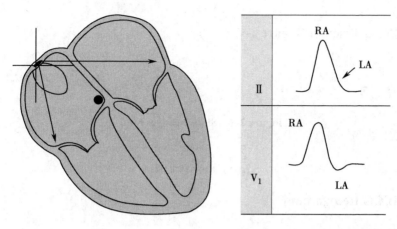

Figure 2-5　Compositions of sinus P wave.

appears small and rounded in lead Ⅱ, and biphasic in lead V₁. Lead Ⅱ and lead V₁ are regarded as the best leads to analyze the electrical activities of both atria on ECG.

Abnormality in Voltage of Sinus P Wave
(Right Atrial Enlargement)

If right atrial enlargement exists, the right atrial depolarization vector which directs anteriorly to the bottom right will increase. The increased depolarization vector is closer to the positive poles of leads Ⅱ, Ⅲ, aVF, causing P waves to be tall and peaked and obviously increased amplitude in leads Ⅱ, Ⅲ, aVF.

[ECG Recognition]

   1. In leads Ⅱ, Ⅲ, aVF, P wave is abnormally tall and peaked, and the voltage exceeds 0.25 mV (P pulmonale).

   2. Electrical axis of P wave often exceeds 70°.

   3. The duration of the P wave is still within normal range.

[ECG Tracing] (Figure 2-6)

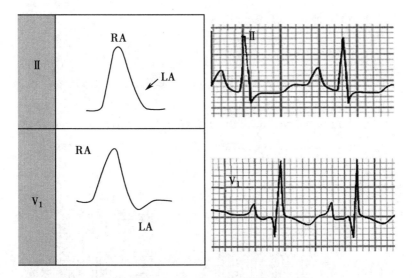

Figure 2-6   Right atrial enlargement.

Abnormality in Duration of Sinus P Wave
(Left Atrial Enlargement)

If left atrial enlargement exists, the prolonged depolarization time will broaden the P wave on ECG. Besides, as a result of the increased left atrial depolarization vector, the resultant atrial depolarization vector points left posteriorly (much closer to the direction of leads I, II, aVR, aVL), and opposite to the direction of lead V_1 on the horizontal plane. This leads to obvious widening of P wave in leads I, II, aVR and aVL, and the widening of negative portion of the P wave in lead V_1 (Figure 2-7).

[ECG Recognition]

1. P wave in leads I, II, aVR, aVL is widened to over 0.12 s (P mitrale).

2. P waves are mostly double-peaked. The second peak is often bigger than that of the first one, and the interspike interval often exceeds 0.04 s.

3. In lead V_1 the voltage of the P wave increases to over 2 mV, and appear biphasic. The terminal negative portion is apparently

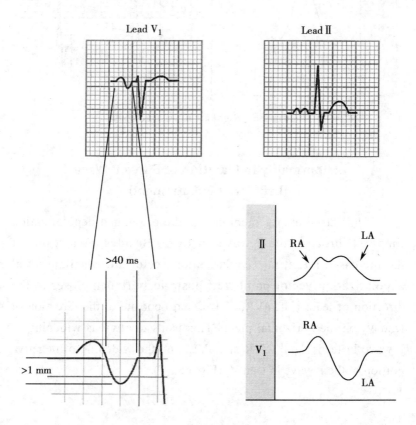

Lead V_1 Lead II

>40 ms

>1 mm

II RA LA

V_1 RA LA

Figure 2-7   Left atrial enlargement.

widened (>40 ms) and deepened (>1 mm), which makes the Ptf-V_1 ⩽−0.04 mm·s (Ptf-V_1 is the terminal vector in lead V_1, the cross product of the negative depth (mm) and duration (s) of the P wave in lead V_1).

[ECG Tracing] (Figure 2-7)

Section 2   Non-sinus P Wave

After the discussion, readers are supposed to understand the characteristics of waveform of the sinus P wave and be able to conduct rough ECG diagnosis using the morphological features of the sinus P wave. Now that sinus P wave exists, non-sinus P wave exists correspondingly. First, let's draw an overview of the morphological features of non-sinus P wave according to those of sinus P wave.

1. Though the P wave is upright in lead Ⅱand inverted in lead aVR, its morphology is different from normal sinus P wave .

2. **Manifestation of non-sinus P wave**: The P wave is inverted in lead Ⅱ and upright in lead aVR. It is generated by the impulse conducted retrogradely from the atrioventricular node, then the atria are excited and the P wave (retrograde P wave) is produced.

I. P Wave Morphologically Different from Normal Sinus P Wave (Atrial P Wave)

Premature Atrial Contraction

The contraction from the atrial ectopic pacemaker that occurs earlier than expectation is called premature atrial contraction. Since it originates in the atrial ectopic pacemaker, different atrial depolarization sequence is produced comparing with sinus pacemaker. As a consequence, P wave generated under this circumstance is different from sinus one, and in order to distinguish them, we use P′ instead.

[ECG Recognition]

1. P′ wave that occurs prematurely is different from sinus P wave morphologically.
2. P′ waves are usually followed by QRS complexes with normal morphology and duration (normal anterograde conduction, Figure 2-8A); a few P′ waves are followed by wide, bizarre QRS complexes (aberrant conduction, Figure 2-8B); a few other P′ waves are followed by no QRS complexes (non-conduction, Figure 2-8C).
3. The P′-R interval is no less than 0.12 s.
4. In most cases the compensatory pause is incomplete.

[ECG Tracing] (Figure 2-8)

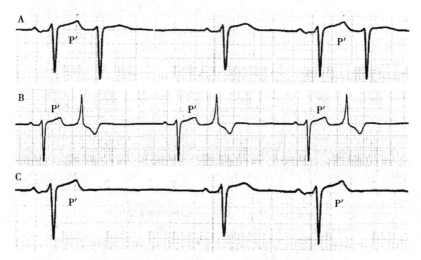

Figure 2-8　Premature atrial contraction.
A. normal anterograde conduction; B. aberrant conduction; C. non-conduction.

Atrial Escape Beat

Escape beat and premature beat are a pair of opposite concepts, the former means the impulses are discharged later than expectation, and the latter comes earlier than expectation. The occurrence of atrial escape beat mainly because: ①the sinus node, for some reason, cannot discharge impulses normally (including the rate of impulses slowing down or asystole); ②the impulses cannot conduct anterogradely due to conduction disturbance; ③other reasons that can cause a long pause. In this case, the downstream ectopic pacemaker will be released from the suppression of normal rates, and discharge impulses in its natural cycles. When only 1 or 2 impulses are discharged by them, it is called escape beat, and if 3 or more are discharged consecutively, it is called escape rhythm.

According to different sites of origin, there are atrial escape beat (rare, Figure2-9), junctional escape beat (the most common type, discussed in detail in section 3 of Chapter 2, Figure 2-15), and ventricular escape beat (common, discussed in detail in Chapter 4).

[ECG Recognition]

1. P′ appears after a long pause and is different from the sinus P wave morphologically.
2. The P′-R interval is no less than 0.12 s.
3. P′ is followed by QRS complexes of normal morphology and duration; wide, bizarre QRS complexes are rare.
4. It is called atrial escape beat if there are 1 to 2 abnormal beats discussed above; it is called atrial escape rhythm if 3 or more such beats are seen in a row, and the rate normally ranges between 50 and 60 bpm.

[ECG Tracing] (Figure 2-9)

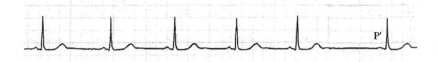

Figure 2-9 Atrial escape beat.

II. Non-sinus P Wave (Retrograde P′ wave)

Premature Atrial Contraction

Ectopic pacemaker located in lower part of the atrium discharges impulses ahead of time, and produces retrograde P′ waves (Figure 2-10).

[ECG Recognition]

1. Retrograde P′ wave which occurs ahead of time and precedes QRS complexes.
2. Usually P′ waves are followed by QRS complexes of normal morphology and duration (normal anterograde conduction); a few P′ waves are followed by wide, bizarre QRS complexes (aberrant conduction); a few other P′ waves are followed by no QRS complexes (non-conduction).
3. The P′-R interval is no less than 0.12 s.
4. Usually the compensatory pause is incomplete.

[ECG Tracing] (Figure 2-10)

Premature Junctional Contraction

The impulse discharged ahead of time by the ectopic pacemaker at the atrioventricular junction is called premature junctional contraction. The junctional impulse which appears early is able to

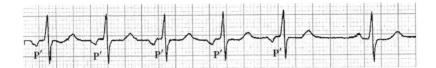

Figure 2-10   Premature atrial contraction with retrograde P' waves.

conduct anterogradely and retrogradely at the same time. Retrograde conduction activates the atria and subsequently produces retrograde P' waves, while anterograde conduction activates the ventricles and produce QRS complexes. Due to different velocities of retrograde and anterograde conduction, the retrograde P' wave may present before (Figure 2-11A) or after the QRS complexes (Figure 2-11B). Based mainly on the P'-R interval and whether the compensatory pause is complete, we can distinguish the premature junctional contraction from the premature atrial contraction when retrograde P' wave precedes the QRS complex. If the P'-R interval is no less than 0.12 s and the compensatory pause is not complete, it is premature atrial contraction; if P'-R interval less than 0.12 s with a complete compensatory pause, it is premature junctional contraction.

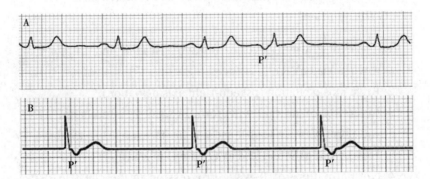

Figure 2-11   Premature junctional contraction.
A: retrograde P' waves appear before the QRS complexes; B: retrograde P' waves appear after the QRS complexes.

[ECG Recognition]

1. QRS complexes that occur ahead of time usually have normal morphology, or sometimes become bizarre as a result of aberrant intraventricular conduction.
2. The retrograde P′ wave may appear before the QRS complex (the P′-R interval is less than 0.12 s in adults, no more than 0.10 s in children, or differs largely from the sinus P-R interval), after the QRS complex (the P′-R interval <0.20 s), or be buried in the QRS complex and difficult to distinguish (absent P wave).
3. Usually the compensatory pause is complete.

[ECG Tracing] (Figure 2-11)

Weird Retrograde P′ Wave (LA/RA Reversal)

When you are reading an ECG and find P′wave (that is, inverted P wave in lead Ⅱ and upright P wave in lead aVR), you are supposed to consider that misplacement of left arm and right arm leads could possibly happen, besides junctional premature contraction.

[ECG Recognition]

1. Apparent P′ wave (inverted P wave in lead Ⅱ and upright P wave in lead aVR).
2. Right axis deviation (pseudo-right axis deviation).
3. Inversion of normal waveform in lead Ⅰ, interchange of waveform between lead Ⅱ and lead Ⅲ, interchange of waveform between lead aVR and lead aVL, normal in lead aVF.
4. Normal pattern of R-wave progression in the chest leads (gradual progression of R wave and regression in S wave from V_1 to V_6).

[ECG Tracing] (Figure 2-12)

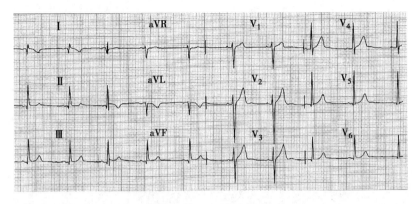

Figure 2-12   LA/RA reversal.

Another Weird Retrograde P′ Wave

Finally, there is yet another possibility for a retrograde P′ wave, congenital dextrocardia. The key to differentiation of dextrocardia from LA/RA Reversal is the pattern of R-wave progression in the chest leads (in the case of dextrocardia, QRS complex shows an rS pattern in all chest leads and regression in amplitude from V_1 to V_6). If retrograde P′ wave shows up with normal R-wave progression, the diagnosis of LA/RA reversal could be made. Retrograde P′ wave with disturbed R-wave progression reveals dextrocardia.

[ECG Recognition]

1. Apparent P′ wave (inverted P wave in lead II and upright P wave in lead aVR).
2. Right axis deviation.
3. Inversion of normal waveform in lead I, interchange of waveform between lead II and lead III, interchange of waveform between lead aVR and lead aVL, normal in lead

aVF.

4. Disturbed R-wave progression (QRS complex shows an rS pattern in all chest leads and regression in amplitude from V_1 to V_6).

[ECG Tracing](Figure 2-13)

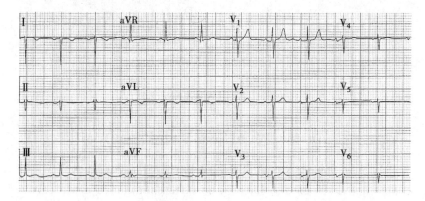

Figure 2-13　Dextrocardia.

Section 3　P Wave Absence

In some cases, junctional premature contraction impulses could only move anterogradely, and could not be conducted backwards. ECG tracing shows an absence of P wave before and after the QRS complex.

[ECG Recognition]

1. Premature QRS complex with normal or bizarre morphology resulting from aberrant ventricular conduction.

2. Absence of P wave before and after QRS complex (retrograde P′ wave is buried in the QRS complex and therefore unidentifiable).

[ECG Tracing] (Figure 2-14)

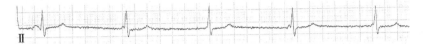

II

Figure 2-14　Absence of retrograde P' wave in junctional premature contraction.

Junctional Escape Beat

Junctional escape beat is defined as escape beat which originates from the junction of atria and ventricles (Figure 2-15).

[ECG Recognition]

1. QRS complex with normal morphology and duration appears after a relatively long pause.
2. Absence of P wave or relevant P wave before most QRS complexes in escape beat. However, presence of retrograde P' wave could be discovered before or after few QRS complexes, in which case, P'-R interval is less than 0.12 s if the retrograde P' wave is before QRS complex, and R-P' interval is less than 0.2 s if it is after.

[ECG Tracing]

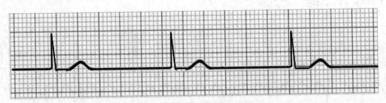

Figure 2-15　Junctional escape beat without retrograde P'.

Atrial Flutter

Atrial flutter is a fast heart rhythm. The main characteristic of atrial flutter is that P waves disappear from ECG tracing in each lead, and are replaced by flutter waves (F waves). Atrial flutter is usually instable. It can be restored to a sinus rhythm, or develop into atrial fibrillation and some cases of atrial flutter can last for quite a time.

[ECG Recognition]

1. P waves disappear from all leads, and are replaced by F waves.
2. F waves have a wave like or saw-toothed appearance, with uniform sizes and F-F interval.
3. F waves usually have a frequency of 250 to 350 bpm.
4. F:R ratio is usually 2:1, so ventricular rate is 140 to 160 bpm.
5. QRS complex is usually normal, but can manifest aberrant ventricular conduction, especially when the conduction ratio appears to be 2:1 and 4:1 alternatively; the heart beat which appeared in the long-short cardiac cycle might be easy to show intraventricular aberrant conduction.

[ECG Tracing] (Figure 2-16)

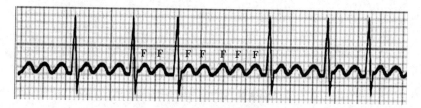

Figure 2-16   Atrial flutter.

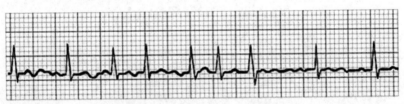

Atrial Fibrillation

Atrial fibrillation is a heart rhythm even faster than atrial flutter. Its main ECG feature is that P waves from each lead disappear and are replaced by small fibrillatory waves (f waves).

[ECG Recognition]

1. P waves disappear from every lead, replaced by f waves.
2. Fibrillatory waves are not uniform in size, appearance nor interval, with a frequency of 450 to 600 bpm.
3. R-R intervals are uneven.
4. Ventricular rate usually increases, but do not exceed 160 bpm. It can be slowed down after administration of digitalis or during chronic atrial fibrillation.
5. QRS complex is normal, but because of the big fluctuation of ventricular cycle, the heart beat which appeared in the long-short cardiac cycle might be easy to show intraventricular aberrant conduction.

[ECG Tracing] (Figure 2-17)

Figure 2-17   Atrial fibrillation.

Sinus Arrest

Sinus arrest is also known as sinus pause, during which SA nodes stop generating electrical impulses due to certain reasons in a period of time, causing the atria or the entire heart to stop functioning.

During this time, lower patent pacemakers usually discharge in place of the SA node, presenting an escape beat or rhythm.

[ECG Recognition]

1. A long interval (P-P interval) appears in a regular sinus rhythm.

2. The long interval does not form a fixed ratio with the normal sinus P-P interval.

3. The long interval is usually followed by an escape beat or rhythm.

[ECG Tracing] (Figure2-18)

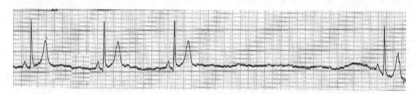

Figure 2-18   Sinus arrest.

Section 4   Common Types of Tachycardia with Narrow QRS Complex

Tachycardia with narrow QRS complex have a QRS interval less than or equal to 120 ms, and a frequency greater than or equal to 100 bpm. 95% of the cases are supraventricular tachycardia, which originates from above the division of the bundle branches; 5% are ventricular tachycardia, particularly idiopathic ventricular tachycardia in children which can have a QRS interval less than 120 ms. Common types of narrow QRS complex tachycardia include atrioventricular nodal reentrant tachycardia (AVNRT), atrioventricular reentrant tachycardia (AVRT) and atrial tachycardia.

Atrioventricular Nodal Reentrant Tachycardia

The structural basis of AVNRT is the two types of conduction pathways with different properties in the AV node, which is called dual atrioventricular nodal pathway. One of the pathways has a slow conduction rate and short refractory period, called slow pathway (α pathway). The other pathway has a fast conduction rate, but longer refractory period, and is known as fast pathway (β pathway). Normally, an excitation originating in the SA node reaches the ventricle via the fast pathway. On reaching the end of the circuit, the excitation go in retrograde via the slow pathway, offsetting the excitation that went in anterograde fashion through the same pathway (Figure 2-19A). When atrial pacemaker discharges an impulse, as fast pathway has a longer refractory period than slow pathway, the impulse more than often pass along the slow pathway which has recovered from the refractory state, resulting in a long P'-R interval. At this time, if the excitation through the fast pathway already nears the end

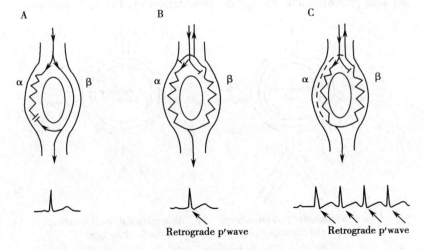

Figure 2-19　Mechanism of slow and fast AVNRT.

of the circuit and the cells in the fast pathway has recovered from the refractory state, the impulse can go in retrograde via the fast pathway back to the atria, but as the same impulse proceed again toward the ventricle, the slow pathway is still in the refractory period, stopping the impulse from passing through again. Therefore, a small pseudo r wave appears on ECG (retrograde P′ wave, Figure 2-19B). The earlier the atria is excited, the slower the excitation pass through the slow pathway, as the impulse reaches the start of the circuit again via the fast pathway as the retrograde limb, the slow pathway has recovered from the refractory state, enabling the impulse to pass through again, forming a continuous reentrant excitation and causing what we call AVNRT (Figure 2-19C). This is the most common mechanism of AVNRT, also known as 'slow-fast'VNRT.

There is another type of AVNRT which is more uncommon. Its fast pathway has a refractory period shorter than the slow pathway. The antergrade conduction of the reentrant excitation is through the fast pathway, and retrograde conduction via the slow pathway,

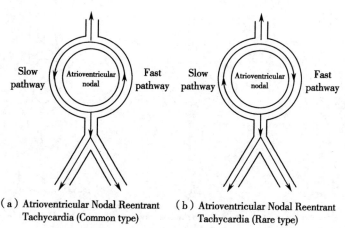

(a) Atrioventricular Nodal Reentrant　　　(b) Atrioventricular Nodal Reentrant
　　　Tachycardia (Common type)　　　　　　　　Tachycardia (Rare type)

Figure 2-20　Two types of AVNRT.

forming 'fast-slow' AVNRT. This type of AVNRT is very rare and makes up approximately 10% of all cases. It is more commonly seen in children. We will not go over the details of the uncommon type (Figure 2-20) and will focus on the 'slow-fast' AVNRT (Figure 2-21) in this chapter.

Slow-Fast Atrioventricular Nodal Reentrant Tachycardia

[ECG Recognition]

1. Tachycardia is usually induced by premature atrial contraction, frequency at 160-200 bpm.
2. R-R intervals are even, heart rhythm is regular.
3. In most cases there are no P waves because the retrograde P wave is buried in QRS complex. In a few cases there might be a retrograde P′ wave after QRS complex, some of which appear at the J point on QRS, forming a pseudo S wave in leads Ⅱ, Ⅲ, aVF and a pseudo R wave in lead V_I.
4. R-P′ interval<P′-R interval, R-P′ interval < 70 ms.
5. QRS complex usually have a normal appearance. If there is aberrant ventricular conduction or existing bundle branch block, QRS complex may appear to be widened. In some patients electrical alternans in the QRS complex might be seen.

[ECG Tracing]

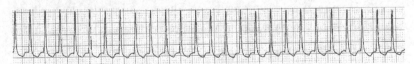

Figure 2-21　Slow-fast atrioventricular nodal reentrant tachycardia.

Atrioventricular Reentrant Tachycardia, AVRT

Under normal circumstances, AV node-His-Purkinje system is the only conduction pathway between the atria and the ventricles. The atrioventricular ring surrounding the system is insulated, functioning as a barrier. In some patients with congenital developmental anomalies, there are additional conduction bundles (also known as accessory pathways) beside the normal conduction pathway. Excitation from the atria can reach the ventricles through the original pathway or the accessory pathway. Because of the unique electrophysiological characteristics of the accessory pathway, atrioventricular reentrant conduction is more likely to occur as the atria, the original atrioventricular conduction pathway, the ventricles as well as the accessory pathways join to form a big reentrant circuit, resulting in AVRT.

There are two types of accessory atrioventricular pathways that cause AVRT:

① Concealed accessory pathway: There can only be retrograde conduction through the pathway and no anterograde conduction, so during a sinus rhythm or tachycardia, impulse is conducted in the normal manner to the ventricles, and passes back through the accessory pathway. Its ECG features include a normal QRS complex with no delta wave (refer to Chap. 3 Sec.2 for pre-excitation syndrome related material). This is called orthodromic AVRT.

② Dominant accessory pathway: There can be both anterograde and retrograde conduction through the pathway. During a sinus rhythm, the sinus excitation can either be conducted in the normal manner down to the ventricles or pass through the accessory pathway and reach some parts of the ventricles at a faster rate, causing associated cardiac muscle cells to depolarize earlier. Its manifestation on the ECG is a delta wave before the QRS complex. When tachycardia occurs, the excitation can spread downward through the normal pathway, go in reverse through the accessory pathway, causing orthodromic AVRT, with normal QRS complex on ECG tracing without any delta wave (Figure 2-22A). The excitation can also spread downward through the accessory pathway and pass back through the normal pathway, causing antidromic AVRT, with wide QRS complex along with delta wave on ECG tracing (Figure 2-22B).

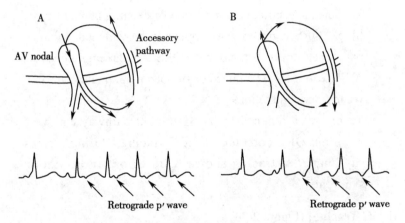

Figure 2-22   AVRT by dominant accessory pathway.

Orthodromic Atrioventricular Reentrant Tachycardia

[ECG Recognition]

1. Heart rate during tachycardia is 150-250 bpm, but it's usually >200 bpm.
2. Regular heart rate.
3. Under most circumstances there is no P wave because the retrograde P wave is buried in the QRS complex, but

occasionally we can see a retrograde P′ wave after the QRS complex.

4. R-P′ interval<P′-R interval, R-P′ interval>70 ms.

5. Atrioventricular conduction ratio is 1 : 1. There shouldn't be atrioventricular block because normal conduction between the atria and the ventricles is the prerequisite for maintaining reentry. If atrioventricular block occurs, we can eliminate the possibility of AVRT.

6. QRS complex usually have a normal appearance. If there is aberrant ventricular conduction or existing bundle branch block, QRS complex may appear to be widened. In some patients electrical alternans in the QRS complex might be seen.

7. AVRT can often be induced or stopped by premature atrial or ventricular contraction.

8. Tachycardia induced by the dominant pathway can have a normal QRS complex on ECG tracing. During a sinus rhythm, ECG tracing shows features of pre-excitation syndrome.

[ECG Tracing] (Figure 2-23)

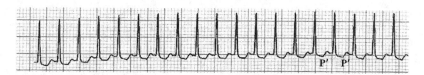

Figure 2-23   **Orthodromic atrioventricular reentrant tachycardia.**

Antidromic Atrioventricular Reentrant Tachycardia

[ECG Recognition]

1. Delta wave can be seen at the start of the QRS complex.
2. Heart rate during tachycardia is between 150 and 250 bpm, usually >200 bpm, with a regular heart rhythm.
3. In most cases there is no P wave. If there is a P′ wave, then the R-P′ interval>P′-R interval.
4. During a sinus rhythm, QRS complex shows features of pre-excitation syndrome.

[ECG Tracing] (Figure 2-24)

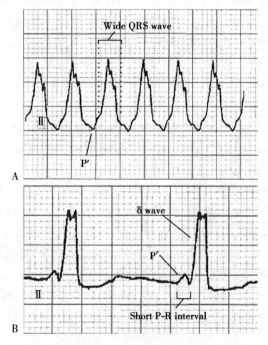

Figure 2-24   Antidromic atrioventricular reentrant tachycardia.
A: during tachycardia; B:during normal sinus rhythm.

Atrial Tachycardia

The mechanism of atrial tachycardia is rather different according to what we see on ECG. It can be categorized into three types, automatic atrial tachycardia (AAT), reentrant atrial tachycardia and multifocal atrial tachycardia (MAT). Its most important characteristic is P waves with altered appearance compared with those from sinus origin.

[ECG Recognition]

1. Atrial rate is usually 150-200 bpm, ventricular rate is usually between 100 and 150 bpm.
2. P wave alter in appearance from those in a normal sinus rhythm (upright in leads Ⅱ, Ⅲ, aVF, inverted in aVR). It can also become a retrograde p′ wave (inverted in leads Ⅱ, II, aVF and upright in aVR). Those with uneven P′-P′ or P′-R intervals are called multifocal atrial tachycardia (MAT).
3. Often, second-degree AV block type I or type Ⅱ can be seen, with a conduction ratio of 2:1, but it does not affect the state of tachycardia.
4. The isoelectric line still exists between P waves (which is distinct from atrial flutter, when the isoelectric line disappears).
5. Stimulation of the vagus nerve cannot stop tachycardia, instead it can aggravate AV block.
6. Heart rate gradually increases at the onset of atrial tachycardia.

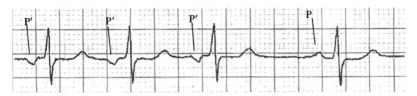

[ECG Tracing] (Figure 2-25)

Figure 2-25   Atrial tachycardia.

Addendum: Algorithm for Differential Diagnosis of QRS Narrow Tachycardia (Figure 2-26)

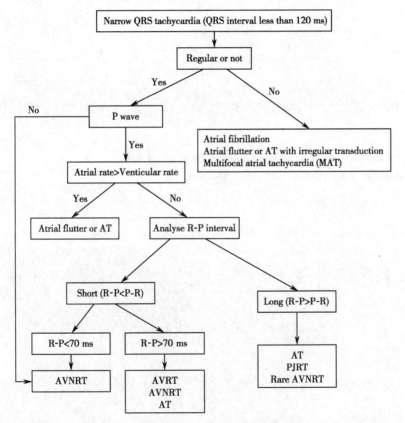

Figure 2-26   Algorithm for differential diagnosis of QRS narrow tachycardia.

Section 5   ECG Practice Strips

Strip 2-1   Rhythm (Regular   Irregular)   Rate (bpm)
Analyze   P wave (Sinus   Non-sinus   Absence)

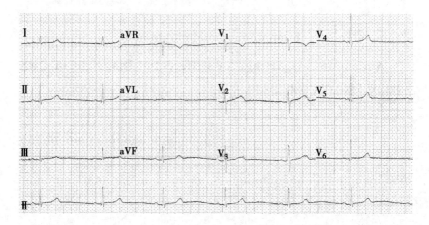

Strip 2-2   Rhythm (Regular   Irregular)   Rate (bpm)
Analyze   P wave (Sinus   Non-sinus   Absence)

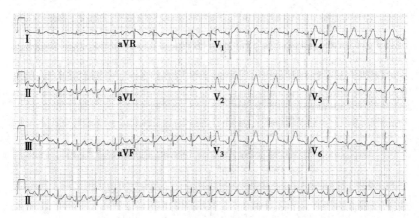

Strip 2-3 Rhythm (Regular   Irregular)   Rate (bpm)

Analyze   P wave (Sinus   Non-sinus   Absence)

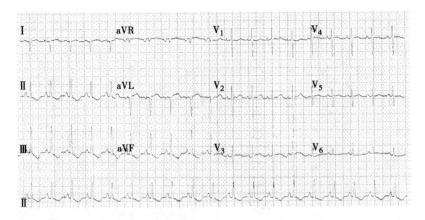

Strip 2-4 Rhythm (Regular   Irregular)   Rate (bpm)

Analyze   P wave (Sinus   Non-sinus   Absence)

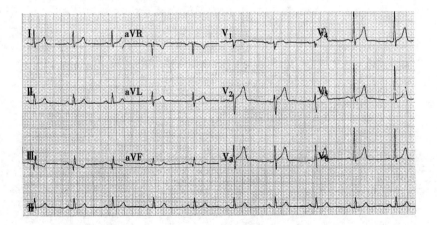

Strip 2-5 Rhythm (Regular   Irregular)   Rate (bpm)

Analyze   P wave (Sinus   Non-sinus   Absence)

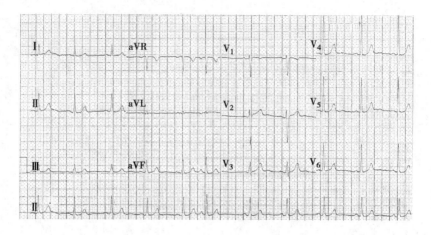

Strip 2-6 Rhythm (Regular   Irregular)   Rate (bpm)

Analyze   P wave (Sinus   Non-sinus   Absence)

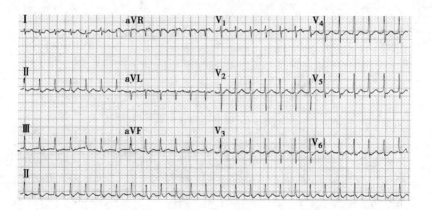

Strip 2-7   Rhythm (Regular   Irregular)   Rate (bpm)

Analyze   P wave (Sinus   Non-sinus   Absence)

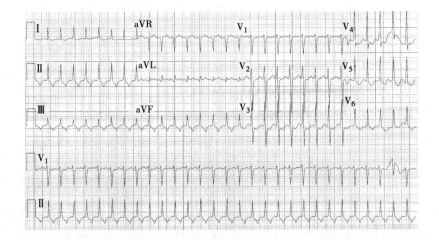

Strip 2-8   Rhythm (Regular   Irregular)   Rate (bpm)

Analyze   P wave (Sinus   Non-sinus   Absence)

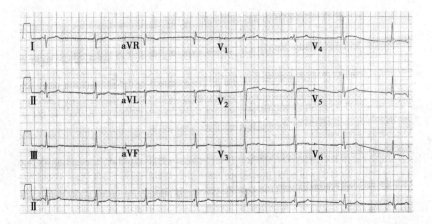

Strip 2-9　Rhythm (Regular　Irregular)　Rate (　　bpm)

Analyze　P wave (Sinus　Non-sinus　Absence)

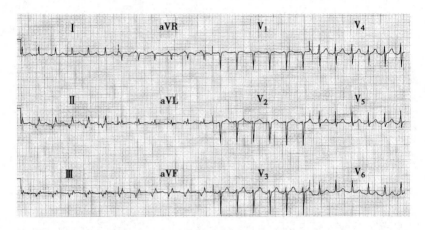

Strip 2-10　Rhythm (Regular　Irregular)　Rate (　　bpm)

Analyze　P wave (Sinus　Non-sinus　Absence)

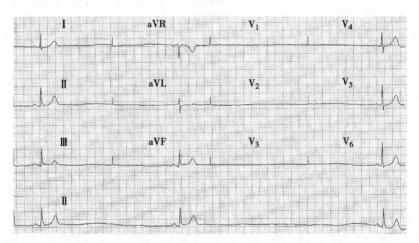

Strip **2-11**   Rhythm (Regular   Irregular)   Rate (bpm)

Analyze   P wave (Sinus   Non-sinus   Absence)

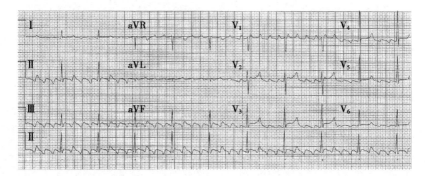

Strip **2-12**   Rhythm (Regular   Irregular)   Rate (bpm)

Analyze   P wave (Sinus   Non-sinus   Absence)

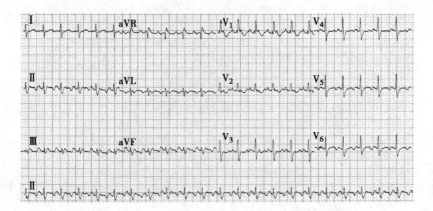

Strip 2-13 Rhythm (Regular Irregular) Rate (bpm)

Analyze P wave (Sinus Non-sinus Absence)

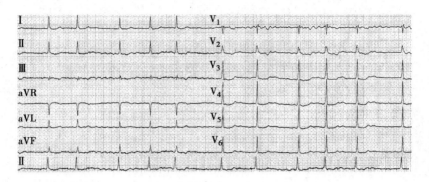

Strip 2-14 Rhythm (Regular Irregular) Rate (bpm)

Analyze P wave (Sinus Non-sinus Absence)

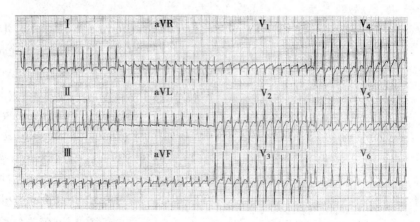

Strip 2-15   Rhythm (Regular   Irregular)   Rate (bpm)
Analyze   P wave (Sinus   Non-sinus   Absence)

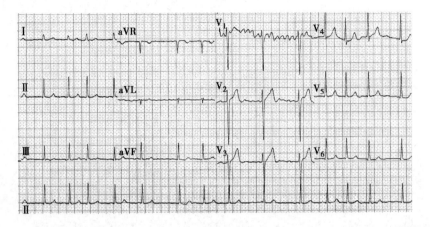

Strip 2-16   Rhythm (Regular   Irregular)   Rate (bpm)
Analyze   P wave (Sinus   Non-sinus   Absence)

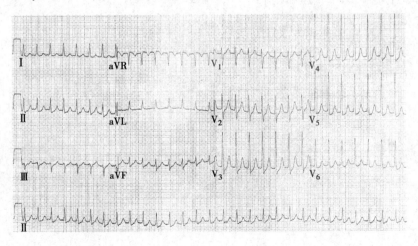

Strip **2-17** Rhythm (Regular　Irregular)　Rate (　　bpm)

Analyze　P wave (Sinus　Non-sinus　Absence)

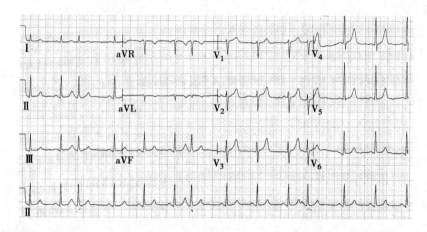

Strip **2-18** Rhythm (Regular　Irregular)　Rate (　　bpm)

Analyze　P wave (Sinus　Non-sinus　Absence)

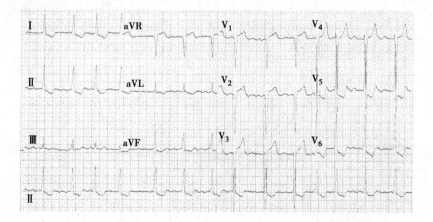

Answers to the Strips

Strip 2-1   Rhythm: Regular   Rate: Less than 60 bpm

Analyze P wave: Sinus P wave

Diagnosis: Sinus bradycardia

Strip 2-2   Rhythm: Regular   Rate: More than 100 bpm

Analyze P wave: Sinus P wave

Diagnosis: Sinus tachycardia

Strip 2-3   Rhythm: Regular   Rate: More than 100 bpm

Analyze P wave: Sinus P wave

Diagnosis: Sinus tachycardia, right atria enlargement

Strip 2-4   Rhythm: Regular   Rate: 60-100 bpm

Analyze P wave: Sinus P wave

Dianosis: Sinus rhythm, normal ECG

Strip 2-5   Rhythm: Irregular   Rate: 60-100 bpm

Analyze P wave: Sinus P wave

Diagnosis: Sinus rhythm, premature atrial contraction

Strip 2-6   Rhythm: Regular   Rate: More than 100 bpm

Analyze P wave: Non-sinus P wave

Diagnosis: Supraventricular tachycardia (AVNRT)

Strip 2-7   Rhythm: Regular   Rate: More than 100 bpm

Analyze P wave: Non-sinus P wave

Diagnosis: Superaventricular tachycardia (AVRT)

Strip 2-8   Rhythm: Irregular   Rate: Less than 60 bpm

Analyze P wave: Sinus P wave

Diagnosis: Sinus bradycardia, junctional escape beat,

complete interference atrioventricular dissociation

Strip 2-9   Rhythm: Regular   Rate: More than 100 bpm

Analyze P wave: Non-sinus P wave

Diagnosis: Atrial tachycardia

Strip 2-10　Rhythm: Irregular　Rate: Less than 60 bpm

Analyze P wave: Sinus P wave

Diagnosis: Sinus arrest

Strip 2-11　Rhythm: Regular　Rate: 60-100 bpm

Analyze P wave: Absence of P wave

Diagnosis: Atrial flutter (with 4 : 1 conduction)

Strip 2-12　Rhythm: Regular　Rate: More than 100 bpm

Analyze P wave: Absence of P wave

Diagnosis: Atrial flutter (with 2 : 1 conduction)

Strip 2-13　Rhythm: Irregular　Rate: 60-100 bpm

Analyze P wave: Absence of P wave

Diagnosis: Atrial fibrillation

Strip 2-14　Rhythm: Regular　Rate: More than 100 bpm

Analyze P wave: Absence of P wave

Diagnosis: Atrial flutter (with 1 : 1 conduction)

Strip 2-15　Rhythm: Irregular　Rate: 60-100 bpm

Analyze P wave: Absence of P wave

Diagnosis: Atrial fibrillation

Strip 2-16　Rhythm: Regular　Rate: More than 100 bpm

Analyze P wave: Non-sinus P wave

Diagnosis: Supraventricular tachycardia

Strip 2-17　Rhythm: Irregular　Rate: 60-100 bpm

Analyze P wave: Sinus P wave

Diagnosis: Sinus rhythm, premature atrial contraction

Strip 2-18　Rhythm: Irregular　Rate: More than 100 bpm

Analyze P wave: Absence of P wave

Diagnosis: Atrial fibrillation, digitalis effect (see Chapter 7), left ventricular hypertrophy (see Chapter 4)

Chapter 3

P-R Interval

The P-R interval is defined as the time between the beginning of the P wave and the beginning of the QRS complex, representing the interval between beginning of depolarization of the atria and the beginning of the ventricles.

Section 1 The Normal P-R Interval

The normal P-R interval is usually between 0.12 and 0.20 s, and it is greatly affected by age and heart rate of the patient. This interval usually decreases with faster heartbeat or in early childhood while increases with slower heartbeat or in old age. Therefore, the normal range of the P-R interval varies with regard to different age and heart rate of the patient (Table 3-1).

Table 3-1 Age, heart rate and maximum of P-R interval(s)

Heart Rate (bpm)	<70	71~90	91~110	111~130	>130
Age(yrs) ≥ 18	0.20	0.19	0.18	0.17	0.16
Age(yrs) 14~17	0.19	0.18	0.17	0.16	0.15
Age(yrs) 7~13	0.18	0.17	0.16	0.15	0.14
Age(yrs) 1.5~6	0.17	0.165	0.155	0.145	0.135
Age(yrs) 0~1.5	0.16	0.15	0.145	0.135	0.125

Section 2 Abnormal P-R Interval

Generally, a prolonged P-R interval longer than 0.20 s is an indication of delayed conduction from the atria to the ventricles, and the patient is said to have atrioventricular block with different causes; shortened P-R interval less than 0.12 s on the other hand, is an indication of enhanced conduction from the atria to the ventricles, which is often seen in preexcitation syndromes.

I. Prolonged P-R Interval (Atrioventricular Block)

Atrioventricular block (AV block, AVB) is the impaired impulse conduction from the atria to the ventricles due to pathologically prolonged refractory period of some parts in the atrioventricular conduction pathways. AV block can mean delayed, incompletely or completely blocked impulse conduction.

The ECG tracing of atrial depolarization is the P wave, while the ventricular depolarization the QRS complexes. Normally, every P wave is followed by a corresponding QRS complex, and the time duration of the P-R interval will not exceed a certain range. When there is an AV block, the ECG shows the association between P wave and the corresponding QRS complexes is abnormal: the P-R interval may prolong, or the corresponding QRS is absent after the P wave.

AV block can be divided into first-degree, second-degree, high-degree and third-degree according to the severity. First-degree, second-degree and high-degree are also known as incomplete AV block, while third-degree is also known as complete AV block.

First-degree AV Block

First-degree AV block is a delay of conduction from the atria to the ventricles, characterized by the P-R interval prolonged over the normal range of the electrocardiogram. However, every supraventricular impulse is able to pass to the ventricles without any dropped beats no matter how long the P-R interval is.

[ECG Recognition]

1. The P-R interval is more than 0.20 s (>0.22 s in the elderly, >0.18 s in children under the age of 14). The P-R intervals are mostly between 0.21 and 0.35 s.

2. The P-R interval is greatly affected by age and heart rate of the patient. Additionally, in patients with first-degree AV block, the P-R interval is longer than the upper limit normal range corresponding to the patient's age group (see Table 3-1).

3. On two continuous electrocardiogram examinations of a patient, the P-R interval is shown to be more than 0.04 seconds longer than that of the previous one without obvious change in the heart rate.

[ECG Tracing] (Figure 3-1)

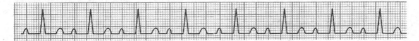

Figure 3-1　First-degree AV block.

Second-degree AV Block

In second-degree AV block, the impulses from the atria to the ventricles are partly interrupted, but not every atrial impulse is able to pass through the AV node to the ventricles, which is defined as dropped beat. As shown in electrocardiogram, not every P wave is followed by a corresponding QRS complex. Second-degree AV block is first described by Wenckebach and MorbitzMorbitz, and therefore it is called Wenckebach and MorbitzMorbitz AV block (type I and type II).

Second-degree AV Block Type I (Mobitz Type I AV Block, Wenckebach Block)

Type I second-degree AV block, also known as Wenckebach block or Mobitz type I AV block, is the most common type in second-degree AV block. Wenckebach block, which is always due to a block within the AV node or in the proximal bundle of His, is mostly a functional block with good prognosis.

[ECG Recognition]

1. The P-R interval is progressively prolonged with each beat until one QRS complex dropped.
2. The P wave is regular sinus P wave.
3. After the dropped QRS complex, item 1 repeats.
4. The ratio of conduction can be fixed or varied; the latter one is more common in clinical practice.

[ECG Tracing] (Figure 3-2)

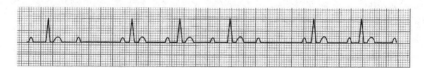

Figure 3-2   Second-degree AV block type I.

Second-degree AV Block Type II (Mobitz Type II Block)

Second-degree AV block type II, also known as the Mobitz type II block, is relatively rare in second-degree AV block. Second-degree AV block type II is mostly an organic disease, or due to a block below the AV node in the distal or branches of bundle of His. Patients with second-degree AV block type II usually have poorer prognosis.

[ECG Recognition]

1. The P-R interval is constant.
2. Regular P wave with abrupt QRS complex drop.
3. The QRS complexes can be normal (if the block happens in distal bundle of His) or resemble the ECG variant of the bundle branch block or fascicular block in morphology (if the block happens in bundle branch).
4. The conduction ratio can be constant or varied.

[ECG Tracing] (Figure 3-3)

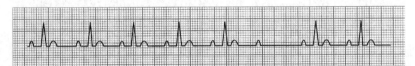

Figure 3-3   Second-degree AV block type II.

High-degree AV Block

Atrioventricular conduction ratio, which means the ratio of P waves to QRS complexes, is often used to measure the severity of AV block. When a tracing shows 4 : 3 block, it means only three out of four atrial impulses are able to pass to the ventricles with one impulse blocked; similarly, 4 : 1 block means only one out of four atrial impulses is able to pass to the ventricles with three impulses blocked. High-degree AV block is identified when two or more successive P wave impulses are not able to reach the ventricles.

[ECG Recognition]

1. The electrocardiogram shows 3 : 1 or greater conduction ratio (e.g. 4 : 1, 5 : 1 or 6 : 1…).

2. As a result of slow ventricular rate, junctional or ventricular escape rhythm are often present (depending on the blocked site), which in electrocardiogram is shown as incomplete AV block.

3. High-degree AV block can be Mobitz type Ⅰ block or Mobitz Type Ⅱ block due to different blocked sites. The blocked sites of Mobitz type Ⅰ block are always within the AV node or, less commonly, in the proximal end of bundle of His, while those of the Mobitz Type Ⅱ block often happens below the AV node in the distal end or branches of bundle of His. Observing P-R interval of the ECG variant of ventricular capture can help distinguish between the two types: constant P-R interval indicates Morbitz type Ⅱ block, while progressive lengthening of P-R interval indicates Morbitz type Ⅰ block.

[ECG Tracing] (Figure 3-4)

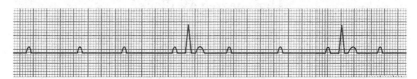

Figure 3-4   High-degree AV block.

Third-degree AV Block

Third-degree AV block is also known as complete AV block. No supraventricular impulses can pass through the AV node to the ventricles. The atria and ventricles are driven by independent pacemakers, resulting in complete AV dissociation. Ventricular capture doesn't exist in third-degree AV block.

[ECG Recognition]

> 1. The P-P intervals and R-R intervals follow to their respective pattern.
>
> 2. P waves and QRS complexes are not related.
>
> 3. P waves appear more frequent than the QRS complexes, because P waves are at sinus rate (60 to 100 bpm) while the QRS complexes are at the junctional (40 to 60 bpm) or ventricular (20 to 40 bpm) escape rate.

[ECG Tracing] (Figure 3-5)

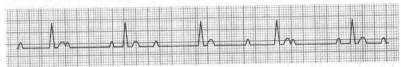

Figure 3-5　Third-degree AV block.

II. Shortened P-R Interval (Preexcitation Syndromes)

The only way by which impulses ordinarily can pass from the atria to the ventricles is through the AV node-His-Purkinje system. In the preexcitation syndromes, there exist abnormal accessory atrioventricular bundles (also known as the accessory pathway or bypass), and atrial impulses can pass through the AV node by the normal pathway or the accessory pathway. On account of the electrophysiological properties of the accessory pathway, the impulses which pass through the bypass can reach the ventricles ahead of time, allowing some or all ventricular myocardial cells to be activated prematurely, and the corresponding electrocardiogram variant is called the ventricular preexcitation. Moreover, the existence of the accessory pathway has made the atrioventricular reentry possible, causing the atrioventricular reentry tachycardia (AVRT). In clinical practice, preexcitation syndrome is defined as ventricular preexcitation with paroxysmal supraventricular tachycardia on the electrocardiogram.

There are two major types of preexcitation syndromes: Wolff-Parkinson-White (WPW) syndrome and Lown-Ganong-Levine (LGL) syndrome.

Wolff-Parkinson-White Syndrome

Wolff-Parkinson-White (WPW) syndrome is also known as the bundle of Kent syndrome. It was first reported by Wolff, Parkinson and White in 1930. In WPW syndrome, the bypass pathway or bundle has been named the bundle of Kent, which is a discrete aberrant conducting pathway located in the atrioventricular ring and connects the atria to ventricles.

[ECG Recognition]

1. The P-R interval is less than 0.12 s.
2. The QRS complex longer than 0.12 s.
3. A preexcitation wave (also known as delta wave) is present at the beginning of the QRS complex.
4. The P-J interval is normal.
5. Secondary ST-T segment abnormality.
6. Some patients may experience recurrent onsets of PSVT.

[ECG Tracing] (Figure 3-6)

WPW syndrome can be roughly divided into type A and type B. In type A preexcitation syndrome, the delta waves in leads V_1 to V_6 are all positive and R waves are predominant in the QRS complex. Type A preexcitation syndrome indicates an accessory pathway located on the left side (Figure 3-7). In type B preexcitation syndrome, the delta waves in leads V_1 to V_3 are either positive or negative, with predominant S waves in the QRS complexes, while

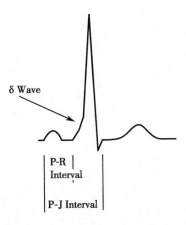

Figure 3-6   Wolff-Parkinson-White syndrome.

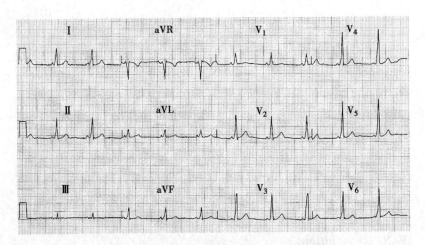

Figure 3-7   Type A preexcitation syndrome.

both the delta waves and QRS are positive in leads V_4 to V_6. Type B preexcitation syndrome indicates an accessory pathway on the right side (Figure 3-8).

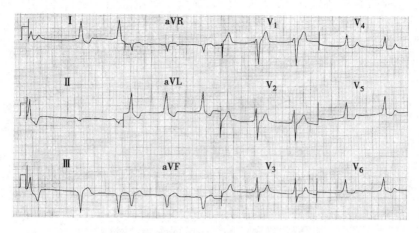

Figure 3-8　Type B preexcitation syndrome.

Lown-Ganong-Levine Syndrome

Lown-Ganong-Levine (LGL) syndrome is characterized by recurrent onsets of tachycardia clinically, while ECG shows only shortening of the P-R interval with normal QRS complexes between episodes of tachycardia (Figure 3-9). It was first reported by Lown, Ganong and Levine in 1952, and therefore designated LGL syndrome. It is also known as the short P-R interval syndrome because its electrical manifestation on ECG is basically the shortening of P-R interval. The existence of aberrant pathways or James fibers within the AV node is the main cause of LGL syndrome.

[ECG Recognition]

1. The P-R interval is less than 0.12 s.
2. The QRS complex is normal without delta waves.
3. Some patients may experience recurrent onsets of tachycardia.

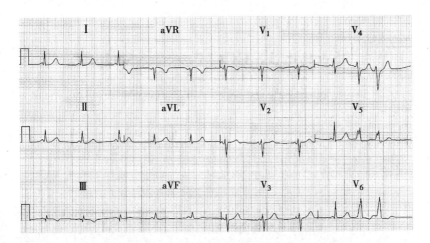

Figure 3-9   Lown-Ganong-Levine syndrome.

[ECG Tracing] (Figure 3-10)

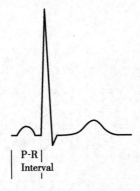

Figure 3-10   Lown-Ganong-Levine syndrome.

Section 3   ECG Practice Strips

Strip 3-1   Rhythm (Regular   Irregular)   Rate (bpm)
P Waves (Sinus   Non-sinus   Absent)
P-R Interval
(Prolonged: Pattern in interval variation   Conduction ratio Relationship between atrial and ventricular depolarization)
(Shortened: Duration and morphology of QRS complex   Delta wave)

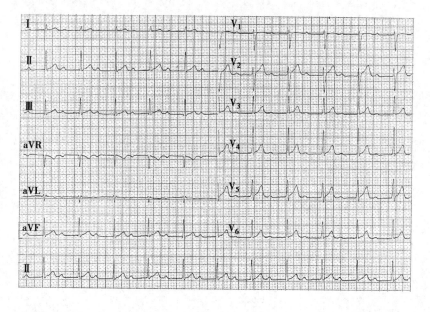

Strip 3-2   Rhythm (Regular   Irregular)   Rate (bpm)
P Waves (Sinus   Non-sinus   Absent)
P-R Interval
(Prolonged: Pattern in interval variation   Conduction ratio Relationship between atrial and
ventricular depolarization)
(Shortened: Duration and morphology of QRS complex   Delta wave)

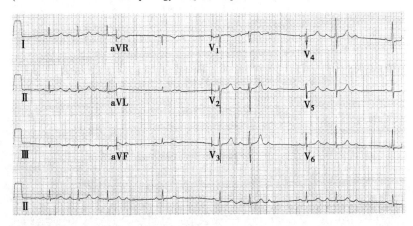

Strip 3-3   Rhythm (Regular   Irregular)   Rate (bpm)
P Waves (Sinus   Non-sinus   Absent)
P-R Interval
(Prolonged: Pattern in interval variation   Conduction ratio Relationship between atrial and
ventricular depolarization)
(Shortened: Duration and morphology of QRS complex   Delta wave)

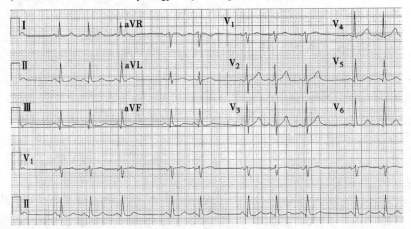

Strip 3-4 Rhythm (Regular Irregular) Rate (bpm)
P Waves (Sinus Non-sinus Absent)
P-R Interval
(Prolonged: Pattern in interval variation Conduction ratio Relationship between atrial and ventricular depolarization)
(Shortened: Duration and morphology of QRS complex Delta wave)

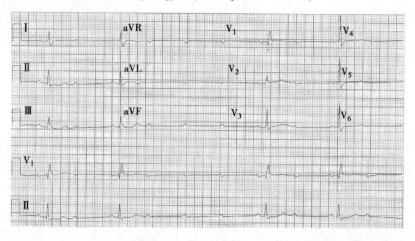

Strip 3-5 Rhythm (Regular Irregular) Rate (bpm)
P Waves (Sinus Non-sinus Absent)
P-R Interval
(Prolonged: Pattern in interval variation Conduction ratio Relationship between atrial and ventricular depolarization)
(Shortened: Duration and morphology of QRS complex Delta wave)

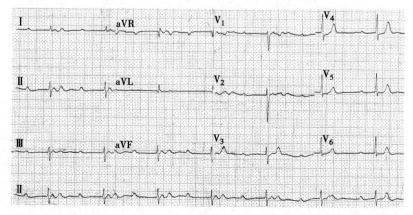

Strip **3-6**   Rhythm (Regular   Irregular)   Rate (bpm)
P Waves (Sinus   Non-sinus   Absent)
P-R Interval
(Prolonged: Pattern in interval variation   Conduction ratio Relationship between atrial and
ventricular depolarization)
(Shortened: Duration and morphology of QRS complex   Delta wave)

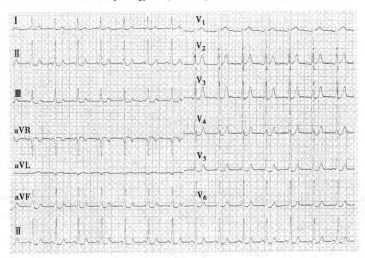

Strip **3-7**   Rhythm (Regular   Irregular)   Rate (bpm)
P Waves (Sinus   Non-sinus   Absent)
P-R Interval
(Prolonged: Pattern in interval variation   Conduction ratio Relationship between atrial and
ventricular depolarization)
(Shortened: Duration and morphology of QRS complex   Delta wave)

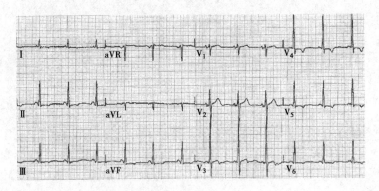

Strip 3-8 Rhythm (Regular   Irregular)   Rate (bpm)

P Waves (Sinus   Non-sinus   Absent)

P-R Interval

(Prolonged: Pattern in interval variation   Conduction ratio Relationship between atrial and ventricular depolarization)

(Shortened: Duration and morphology of QRS complex   Delta wave)

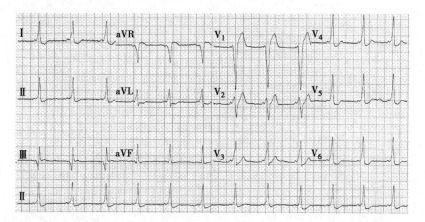

Strip 3-9 Rhythm (Regular   Irregular)   Rate (bpm)

P Waves (Sinus   Non-sinus   Absent)

P-R Interval

(Prolonged: Pattern in interval variation   Conduction ratio Relationship between atrial and ventricular depolarization)

(Shortened: Duration and morphology of QRS complex   Delta wave)

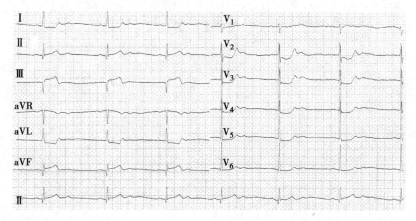

Strip **3-10**   Rhythm (Regular   Irregular)   Rate (bpm)

P Waves (Sinus   Non-sinus   Absent)

P-R Interval

(Prolonged: Pattern in interval variation   Conduction ratio   Relationship between atrial and ventricular depolarization)

(Shortened: Duration and morphology of QRS complex   Delta wave)

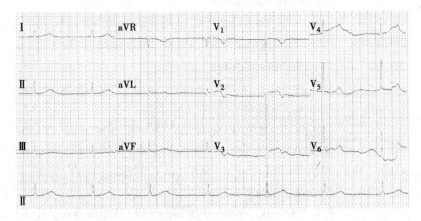

Answers to the Strips

Strip 3-1   Rhythm: Regular   Rate: 60 to 100 bpm

P wave: Sinus P wave

P-R Interval: Prolonged, over 0.21 s

Diagnosis: Sinus rhythm, first-degree AV block

Strip 3-2   Rhythm: Irregular   Rate: 60 to 100 bpm

P wave: Sinus P wave

P-R Interval: Progressively prolonged until QRS complex drop happens

Diagnosis: Sinus rhythm, second-degree AV block type I

Strip 3-3   Rhythm: Irregular   Rate: 60 to 100 bpm

P wave: Sinus P wave

P-R Interval: Constant P-R interval with abrupt QRS complex drop

Diagnosis: Sinus rhythm, second-degree AV block type II

Strip 3-4 Rhythm: Irregular   Rate: 60 to 100 bpm

P wave: Sinus P wave

P-R Interval: P wave is often blocked with occasional successful conduction

Diagnosis: Sinus rhythm, high-degree AV block

Strip 3-5 Rhythm: Regular   Rate: 60 to 100 bpm

P wave: Sinus P wave

P-R Interval: P waves and QRS complexes are not related. Complete AV dissociation

Diagnosis: Third-degree AV block, junctional escape rhythm

Strip 3-6 Rhythm: Regular   Rate: 60 to 100 bpm

P wave: Sinus P wave

P-R Interval: Apparently shortened. Delta wave at the beginning of the QRS complex

Diagnosis: Sinus rhythm, WPW syndrome

Strip 3-7 Rhythm: Regular   Rate: 60 to 100 bpm

P wave: Sinus P wave

P-R Interval: Apparently shortened. No delta wave at the beginning of the QRS complex

Diagnosis: Sinus rhythm, L-G-L syndrome

Strip 3-8 Rhythm: Regular   Rate: 60 to 100 bpm

P wave: Sinus P wave

P-R Interval: Apparently shortened. Delta wave at the beginning of the QRS complex

Diagnosis: Sinus rhythm, WPW syndrome

Strip 3-9 Rhythm: Regular   Rate: 60 to 100 bpm

P wave: Sinus P wave

P-R Interval: Not sure the change of P-R interval (neither

progressively prolonged nor constant P-R interval), every two P waves could only conduct one

Diagnosis: Sinus rhythm, second-degree AV block (2:1 conduction)

Strip 3-10   Rhythm: Regular   Rate: less than 60 bpm

P wave: Sinus P wave

P-R Interval: Prolonged, over 0.21 s (almost 0.8 s)

Diagnosis: Sinus bradycardia, first-degree AV block

Chapter 4

QRS Complex

Section 1　Normal QRS Complex

I. Features of Normal QRS Complex

QRS complex is a group of waves of comparatively deep amplitude, and shows the electrical changes during left and right ventricular depolarization.

The morphological features of normal QRS complex can be summarized into the main wave's direction and the morphology of Q (q) wave.

1. The main wave is positive, in leads I, II and V_4 to V_6; while the main wave is negative in leads aVR, V_1.

2. From lead V_1 to V_6, R wave grows taller, S wave grows lower, and R/S ratio becomes larger

3. In leads V_1 and V_2, there should be no Q (q) wave (QS pattern can be present). In leads aVR, aVL, III, there can be Q or q wave. In leads I, II, aVF, V_4 to V_6, Q wave should not be present (q wave is probably present).

Features of Normal QRS Complex Voltage:

1. In at least one limb lead, the sum of Q, R, S voltages (sum of the absolute values) is greater than or equal to 0.5 mV.

2. In at least one chest lead, the sum of QRS voltages is greater than or equal to 0.8 mV.

3. $R_{V5}<2.5$ mV, $R_{aVL}<1.2$ mV, $R_{aVF}<2.0$ mV, $R_I<1.5$ mV, $R_{V5}+$

S_{V1}<3.5-4.0 mV.

　　4. R_{V1}<1.0 mV, $R_{V1}+S_{V5}$<1.2 mV, R_{aVR}<0.5 mV.

If you think what is mentioned above lengthy or hard to memorize, don't worry and just keep reading, and you will find some simple drawing can help you understand and memorize these details with ease.

II. QRS Vector Loop

Since the myocardial cells participating in depolarization locate in different parts of the heart, the vectors that represent their depolarization can point to different directions, when the ventricles depolarize. The way two vectors interact are: if they have the same direction, they are enhanced; if they have opposite directions, they are weakened; if they form angle between 0° and 180°, the diagonal of the parallelogram is defined as their resultant vector, or mean vector (Figure 4-1). Therefore, the interaction all the vectors have with each other at any moment can be summed into an instant resultant vector.

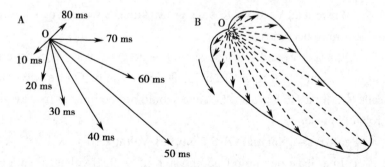

Figure 4-1　Formation of QRS vector loop.

A: Divide the ventricular depolarization into 9 parts, record the amplitude and direction of the instantaneous complex vector; B: Draw a line to connect the termination of the vectors together in proper order and you get a QRS vector loop.

Since the number and the position of the myocardial cells involved in the depolarization are constantly changing, the length and direction of the instant resultant vector vary at different moment of the ventricular depolarization. If we draw a line to connect the termination of the vectors together in an order, or record the process of the changes, we can get a curve, a vector loop in three dimensional spaces (special QRS vector loop).

III. Formation of Normal QRS Complex in Limb Leads

If we placed the QRS vector loop into hexaxial reference system that we've learnt before, we could easily understand the morphology of QRS complex in limb leads (Figure 4-2 to Figure 4-5).

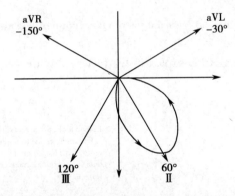

Figure 4-2　Projection of QRS vector loop on axes in hexaxial reference system.

[Formation of QRS complex in lead I] (Figure 4-3)

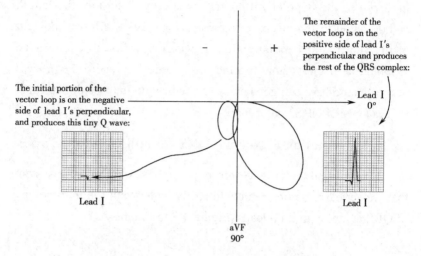

Figure 4-3　Formation of QRS complex in lead I.

[Formation of QRS complex in lead aVF] (Figure 4-4)

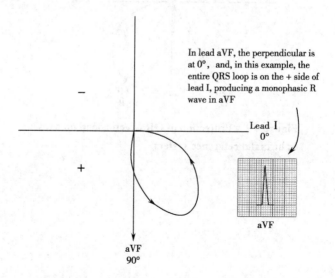

Figure 4-4　Formation of QRS complex in lead aVF.

[Formation of QRS complex in lead III] (Figure 4-5)

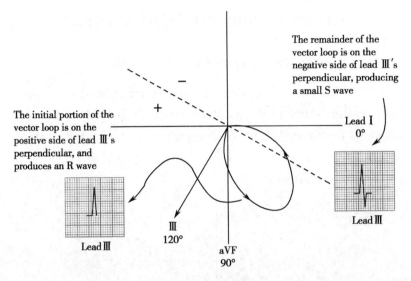

Figure 4-5   Formation of QRS complex in lead III.

Similar to the QRS complex in all limb leads, we can understand QRS complex in all six chest leads when the vectors in QRS vector loop are projected on chest lead axes (Figure 4-6).

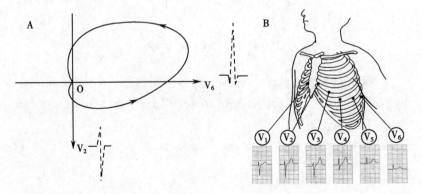

Figure 4-6   QRS vector loop projected on chest leads axes (A) and QRS complex waveform in chest leads (B).

Section 2　Abnormal QRS Complex

I. Abnormalities in QRS Complex Axis

The direction of ECG axis is usually measured by the angle between the axis and the positive direction of lead I axis. The diagnosis recommended by WHO guideline regarding electric axis is as follows:

[Axis Deviation] (Figure 4-7)

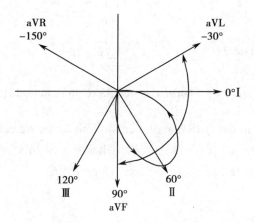

Figure 4-7　Axis deviation.

−30° to +90°, no axis deviation; −30° to −90°, left axis deviation; +90° to +180° right axis deviation; −90° to −180° uncertain axis (axis of 'no man's land')

To determine axis deviation, we should mainly focus on leads I and aVF

No Axis Deviation

[ECG Recognition]

1. The cardiac electric axis lies between −30° and +90°.

2. Two common variants:

① Main wave is positive in both leads Ⅰ and aVF (Figure 4-8A): For the main wave in lead Ⅰ is positive, the QRS axis is in the positive direction of lead Ⅰ axis, that is, in the first or forth quadrant (of the frontal plane). For the main wave in lead aVF is positive, the QRS axis is in the positive direction of lead aVF axis, in other words, in the third quadrant or forth quadrant. Therefore the QRS axis lies in the forth quadrant (0° to +90°). It is no axis deviation.

② The main wave is positive in leads Ⅰ and Ⅱ, and negative in lead aVF (Figure 4-8B): For the main wave in lead Ⅰ is positive, the QRS axis is in the positive direction of lead Ⅰ axis, that is, in the first or forth quadrant; For the main wave in lead aVF is negative, the QRS axis is in the negative direction of lead aVF axis, that is, in the first or second quadrant. Therefore the QRS axis lies in the first quadrant (0° to −90°). Since the main wave is positive in lead Ⅱ, the QRS axis is within 0° to −30°, in other words, it is no axis deviation.

[ECG Tracing] (Figure 4-8)

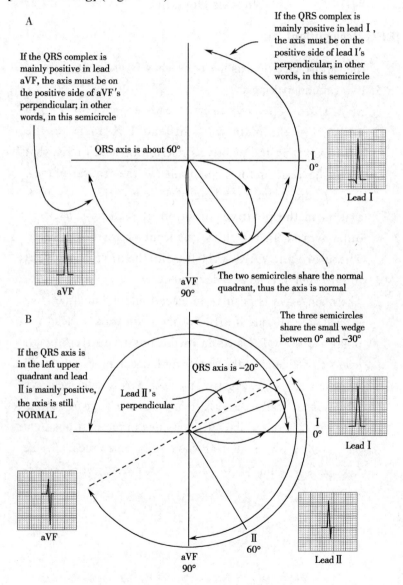

Figure 4-8　Determination of no axis deviation.

A. positive main wave in aVF; B. negative main wave in aVF.

Left Axis Deviation

[ECG Recognition]

1. The angle of cardiac electric axis lies between –30° and –90°.
2. The main wave is positive in lead I , and negative in leads aVF and II. For the main wave in lead I is positive, the QRS axis is in the positive direction of lead I axis, that is, in the first or forth quadrant. For the main wave in lead aVF is negative, the QRS axis is in the negative direction of lead aVF axis, that is, in the first or second quadrant. Therefore, the QRS axis lies in the first quadrant (0° to –90°). Since the main wave is negative in lead II, the QRS axis is within –30° to –90°, in other words, it is left axis deviation.

[ECG Tracing] (Figure 4-9)

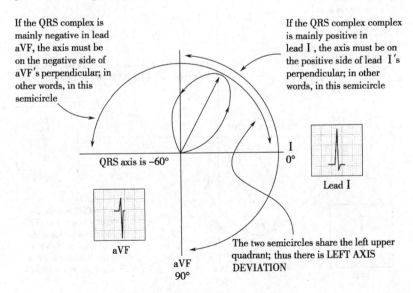

If the QRS complex is mainly negative in lead aVF, the axis must be on the negative side of aVF's perpendicular; in other words, in this semicircle

If the QRS complex complex is mainly positive in lead I , the axis must be on the positive side of lead I 's perpendicular; in other words, in this semicircle

QRS axis is –60°

I
0°

Lead I

aVF

aVF
90°

The two semicircles share the left upper quadrant; thus there is LEFT AXIS DEVIATION

Figure 4-9   Left axis deviation.

Right Axis Deviation

[ECG Recognition]

1. The cardiac electric axis lies between +90° and +180°.

2. The main wave is negative in lead I , and positive in lead aVF. For the main wave in lead I is negative, the QRS axis is in the negative direction of lead I axis, that is, in the second or third quadrant. For the main wave in lead aVF is positive, the QRS axis is in the positive direction of lead aVF axis, that is, in the third or fourth quadrant. Therefore, the QRS axis lies in the third quadrant (+90° to +180°). It is right axis deviation.

[ECG Tracing] (Figure 4-10)

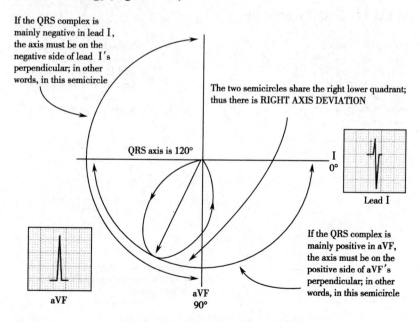

Figure 4-10   Right axis deviation.

Uncertain Axis (No Man's Land)

[ECG Recognition]

1. The cardiac electric axis lies between –90° and –180°.
2. The main wave is negative in leads Ⅰ and aVF. For the main wave in lead Ⅰ is negative, the QRS axis is in the negative direction of lead Ⅰ axis, that is, in the second or third quadrant. For the main wave in lead aVF is negative, the QRS axis is in the negative direction of lead aVF axis, that is, in the first or second quadrant. Therefore, the QRS axis lies in the second quadrant (–90° to –180°). It is uncertain axis.

[ECG Tracing] (Figure 4-11)

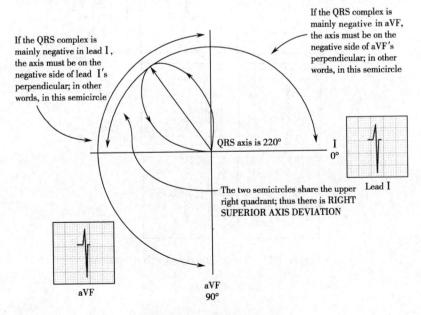

If the QRS complex is mainly negative in lead Ⅰ, the axis must be on the negative side of lead Ⅰ's perpendicular; in other words, in this semicircle

If the QRS complex is mainly negative in aVF, the axis must be on the negative side of aVF's perpendicular; in other words, in this semicircle

QRS axis is 220°

Ⅰ
0°

The two semicircles share the upper right quadrant; thus there is RIGHT SUPERIOR AXIS DEVIATION

Lead Ⅰ

aVF

aVF
90°

Figure 4-11   Uncertain axis.

[The summary of axis deviation] (Figure 4-12)

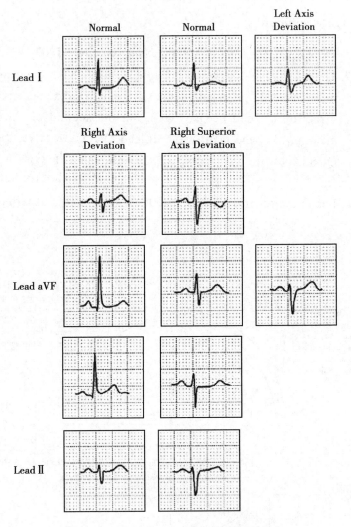

Figure 4-12 The summary of axis deviation.

II. Abnormalities in QRS Complex Voltage

Excess QRS Voltages (High QRS Voltages)

Left Ventricular Hypertrophy

[ECG Recognition]

1. QRS voltage changes: **R_{V5} or R_{V6} voltage is greater than 2.5 mV; $R_{V5}+S_{V1}$ is greater than 4.0** mV (for female is greater than 3.5 mV); R_I voltage is greater than 1.5 mV; $R_I + S_{III}$ is greater than 2.5 mV; R_{aVL} voltage is greater than 1.2 mV or R_{aVF} voltage is greater than 2.0 mV.

2. Prolonged QRS complex duration: QRS complex duration prolonged to 0.10-0.11 s, but still less than 0.12 s.

3. Left axis deviation: Most patients with left ventricular hypertrophy show mild or moderate left axis deviation.

4. Secondary ST-T change: In leads where the R wave predominates in the QRS (such as the left chest leads), the ST segment depression is greater than 0.05 mm with flat, biphasic or inverted T wave; while in the leads where the S wave predominates (such as right chest leads), ST segment elevation can correspondingly appear with tall upright T wave. An increased QRS complex voltage with ST-T change is left ventricular hypertrophy with strain.

[ECG Tracing] (Figure 4-13)

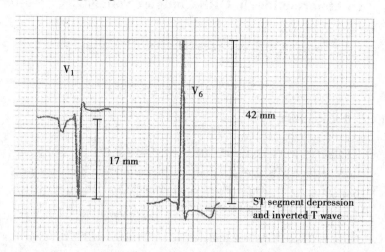

Figure 4-13   Left ventricular hypertrophy.

Right Ventricular Hypertrophy

[ECG Recognition]

1. QRS complex morphology change: QRS complex shows qR pattern in V_1, R/S is greater than 1 in leads V_1 and aVR; R/S is less than 1 in lead V_5; evident clockwise transposition can be seen and QRS complex shows rS pattern from V_1 to V_4, even to V_6 sometimes.

2. QRS complex voltage changes (Figure 4-14): **QRS complex voltage increases: Voltage in R_{V1} is greater than 1.0 mV; $R_{V1}+S_{V5}$ is greater than 1.2 mV; R_{aVR} is greater than 0.5 mV.**

3. Right axis deviation.

4. ST-T Change: ST segment is depressed with biphasic or inverted T wave in V_1. Tall R wave in lead V_1 with ST-T change is defined as right ventricular hypertrophy with strain.

[ECG Tracing] (Figure 4-14)

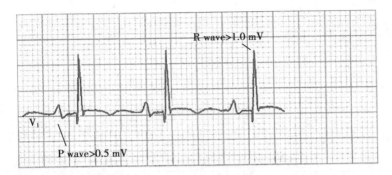

R wave>1.0 mV

V₁

P wave>0.5 mV

Figure 4-14   Right ventricular hypertrophy.

Low Voltage in QRS Complex

Common causes

1. Low voltage caused by myocardium: restrictive cardiomyopathy (amyloidosis, sarcoma, etc).

2. Increased impedance between tissue (myocardium) that forms voltage and leads: fat (overweight), air (COPD, pneumothorax) and water (pericardial or pleural effusion, ascites).

3. Hypothyroidism.

[ECG Recognition]

1. No absolute voltage value of any QRS complexes in any chest leads ≥ 0.8 mV (8mm).

2. Or no absolute voltage value of any QRS complexes in any limb leads ≥ 0.5 mV (known as low voltage in limb leads).

[ECG Tracing] (Figure 4-15)

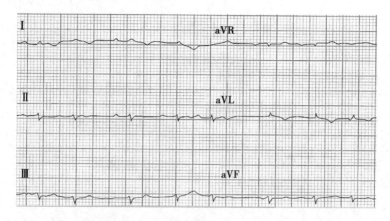

Figure 4-15   Low QRS voltage in limb leads.

III. Wide QRS Complex

Wide QRS complex has a duration greater than 0.12 s. Common causes include premature ventricular contraction, ventricular escape, implantation of artificial cardiac pacemaker, W-PW syndrome, bundle branch or fascicular block. Electrolyte and acid-base balance disturbances may also be included.

Premature Ventricular Contraction(PVC)

[ECG Recognition]

1. QRS complexes have wide (>0.12 s in adults and >0.10 s in children) and bizarre appearance. T wave and QRS complex are in the opposite direction.
2. No corresponding P waves are present before PVC.
3. Retrograde P′ wave may appear after the QRS complex and R-P′ >0.20 s.

4. Usually PVC is followed by a full compensatory pause. However, a non-compensatory pause is also possible.

[ECG Tracing] (Figure 4-16)

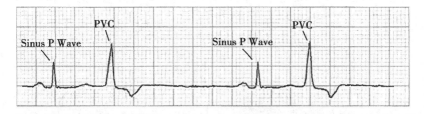

Figure 4-16　Premature ventricular contraction: ventricular bigeminy.

Ventricular Escape

[ECG Recognition]

1. In combination with bradycardia, the delayed QRS wave is wide (>0.12 s in adults and >0.10 s in children) and bizarre. T wave and QRS complex are in the opposite direction.
2. No corresponding P wave is present before the escape beat.

[ECG Tracing] (Figure 4-17)

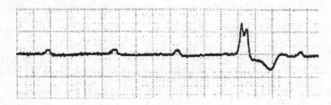

Figure 4-17　Ventricular escape.

ECG Recognition with Artificial Cardiac Pacemakers

An artificial cardiac pacemaker (Figure 4-18) is composed by a power source that generates regular, timed stimuli (heart is stimulated by the electric current which is depicted as spike in ECG) and electrodes (can be classified into unipolar electrode with more stimulation and bipolar electrodes with less stimulation).

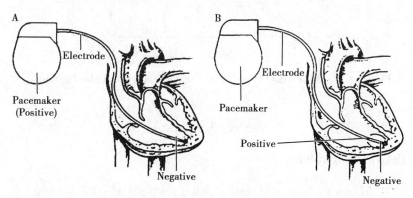

Figure 4-18   Pacemaker with unipolar electrode and pacemaker with bipolar electrode.
A: pacemaker is positive, electrode is negative; B: electrodes have both positive and negative side

According to different principles, pacemakers can be divided into single-chamber pacemaker that has one lead placed in the heart and paces either right atrium or ventricle, dual-chamber pacemaker that has one lead placed in the right atrium and the other in the right ventricle, cardiac resynchronization therapy (CRT) or tri-chamber pacemaker that adds one more lead to the coronary sinus (Figure 4-19).

An international code called NBG code can be used to identify most of the pacemaking system, where A stands for the right atrium, V stands for the right ventricle, D stands for dual, O stands for none, I

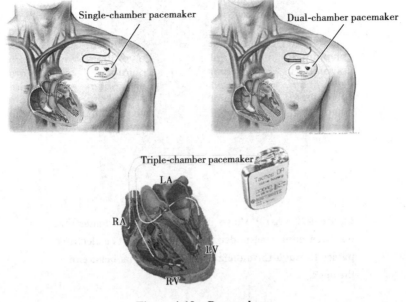

Figure 4-19　Pacemakers.

stands for inhibiting pacing, R stands for triggering pacing.

- The first letter describes the chamber paced (A, V, D).
- The second letter describes the chamber sensed (A, V, D or O).
- The third letter describes the response to sensing (I, R, D or O).
- The forth letter describes the programmable functions.

Right Ventricle Pacemaker

Right ventricle pacemaker, otherwise called ventricular inhibited pacing(VVI), is the most common type of pacemakers, in which the electrode is usually placed in the apex (Figure 4-20). This electrode can sense electrical activities in the right ventricle. If electrical activities by the heart itself are sensed, the pacemaker is inhibited. Otherwise, the pacemaker will pace the ventricle after a pre-set interval.

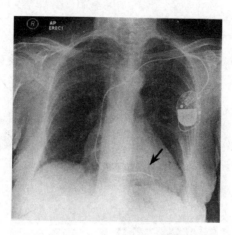

Figure 4-20 X-ray shows right ventricle pacemaker that has been implanted under the left shoulder. The electrode passes through the subclavian vein while its head-end in the apex.

Indications for VVI pacemakers:

- Slow ventricular rates or atrial fibrillation that causes asystole.
- Sino-atrial node diseases.
- Atrial ventricular block.

Drawback: Artificially atrioventricular dyssynchrony.

[ECG Recognition]

1. The spike is followed by a wide QRS complex which resembles left bundle branch block.
2. The pacemaker spike is big in unipolar pacing while small in bipolar pacing.
3. If electrical activities by the heart itself are sensed by the pacemaker, the impulse is inhibited in a pre-set interval. Intermittent pacing will be showed on ECG as non-equal ventricle pacing rhythm and patients'own rhythm.

[ECG Tracing] (Figure 4-21)

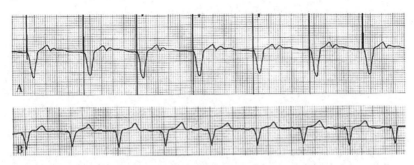

Figure 4-21 Ventricular pacemakers.

A: unipolar pacing in VVI (the pacemaker spike is big); B: bipolar pacing in VVI
(the pacemaker spike is small)

Right Atrium Pacemaker

Right atrium pacemaker is also known as atrial inhibited pacing
(AAI). This is a relatively rare type. The electrode is placed in the
right atrium, usually the right auricle (Figure 4-22, Figure 4-23).
The pacemaker can sense patients' own electrical activities in the
right atrium. If the rate of sinus pulse is higher than the pre-set level,
the pacemaker is inhibited. Otherwise, the pacemaker will work
continuously.

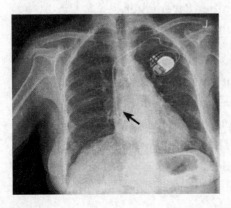

**Figure 4-22 X-ray shows the
right atrium pacemaker that has
been implanted under the left
shoulder. The electrode passes
through the subclavian vein
while its head-end in the right
auricle.**

Indications for AAI pacemakers:

* Sino-atrial node dysfunction without atrial ventricular node diseases.

* Young patients with history of carotid sinus syncope.

Drawback: Not suitable for patients with severe atrial ventricular block.

[ECG Recognition]

1. The spike is followed by a sinus P wave.

2. The P-R interval and QRS complex are usually normal, indicating the atrial ventricular node is functioning well.

3. If the pacemaker can sense patients' own electrical activities, the pacemaker is inhibited during the pre-set interval, showing intermittent pacing on ECG.

[ECG Tracing] (Figure 4-23)

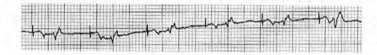

Figure 4-23   Right ventricular pacemaker.

Dual Chamber Pacemaker

Dual chamber pacemaker, otherwise known as DDD pacemaker, is the most common type. It has two electrodes with one in the right atrium and the other in the right ventricle (Figure 4-24, Figure 4-25). Both of the electrodes can sense patients' own electrical activities. If no electrical activities by the patient are sensed, atrium pacing will work in the pre-set interval. The maximum value of P-R interval is also set. If the pacemaker does not sense ventricular electrical activities during the set duration, ventricle pacing will work.

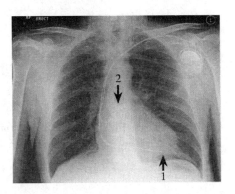

Figure 4-24   X-ray shows DDD
pacemaker that has been implanted
under the left shoulder. The two
electrodes pass through the subclavian
vein. One electrode is placed in the
apex (arrow 1) and the other electrode
is placed in the right auricle (arrow 2).

Indications for DDD pacemaker:

- Sino-atrial node dysfunction.
- Atrial ventricular block.
- Chronic bifascicular block with alternating bundle branch block.
- Carotid sinus hypersensitivity or neurogenic syncope.

Advantage: Guarantee the sequential contraction of the atria and the ventricles.

[ECG Recognition]

1. When the atria and the ventricles are both been pacing, the atrium pacemaker spike is followed by a P wave while the ventricle pacemaker spike is followed by a ventricular pre-excitation wave.
2. When the rate of patients' own atrium pacing is higher than the threshold, the pacemaker is inhibited. When the duration of patients' own P-R interval is larger than the pre-set atrial ventricular interval, ventricle pacing is triggered.
3. If the pacemaker can sense patients' own electrical activities, the pacemaker is inhibited during the pre-set interval, showing intermittent pacing on ECG.

[ECG Tracing] (Figure 4-25)

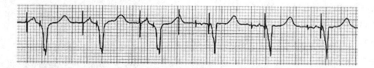

Figure 4-25   Dual chamber pacemaker.

Triple Chamber Pacemaker

Triple chamber pacemaker or cardiac resynchronization therapy (CRT) is also called dual-ventricle pacing (Figure 4-26, Figure 4-27). Patients suffered from severe heart failure, especially those who have left bundle branch block and obviously wide QRS complexes on their ECG, may have imbalance in cardiac synchronization, which decreases the stroke volume and exacerbates heart failure. CRT can make left and right ventricles contract synchronously and improve symptoms caused by heart failure. This is achieved by two electrodes (Figure 4-26). One is placed in the branch of coronary sinus (venous

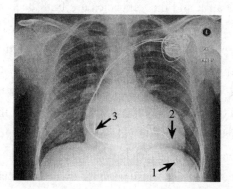

Figure 4-26   X-ray shows CRT pacemaker that has been implanted under the left shoulder. One electrode is placed in the apex (arrow 1), one is placed in the coronary sinus (arrow 2), and the other is placed in the right auricle (arrow 3).

system of coronary circulation, draining into right atrium) to pace the left ventricle while the other is placed in the right ventricle. Besides, there is often another electrode in the right atrium because the atrium contraction may also contribute to cardiac output.

Best indications for CRT:

+ Sinus rhythm.

+ Ventricle ejection fraction is less than 35%.

+ Left bundle branch block with QRS complexes wider than 150 ms.

+ NYHA III to IV with symptoms of heart failure.

Advantage: Guarantee the synchronous contractions in both of the ventricles, improve symptoms caused by heart failure and increase the stroke volume.

[ECG Recognition]

1. Forced dual-ventricle pacing in order to guarantee synchronization. Two ventricular pacemaker spikes are showed on ECG.
2. The following QRS complexes can be narrow left or right bundle branch block pattern.
3. The reason why some patients do not have the electrode in the atrium is that they suffer from atrial fibrillation or flutter.

[ECG Tracing] (Figure 4-27)

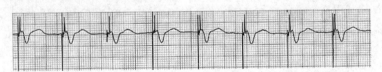

Figure 4-27   Triple chamber pacemaker.

Bundle Branch and Fascicular Block

Right Bundle Branch Block

The sequence of depolarization changes into interventricular septum to the left ventricle to the right ventricle because of right bundle branch block. The end of QRS complex is prolonged with changed pattern (Figure 4-28).

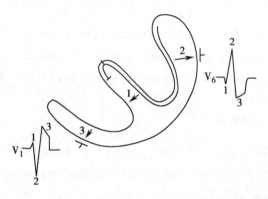

Figure 4-28   The principle of changed pattern in QRS complex in RBBB.

[ECG Recognition]

1. It is complete right bundle branch block when the duration of QRS complexes is greater than or equal to 0.12 s. Otherwise, it is incomplete right bundle branch block.
2. QRS complex resembles rsR′ or 'M' configuration in lead V_1 or V_2.
3. S wave is broad (duration ≥ 0.04 s) and notched in leads Ⅰ, V_5 and V_6.
4. QRS complex resembles QR pattern in lead aVR with wide and notched R wave.

5. The duration of R wave in V_1 is greater than 0.05 s. ST segment is mildly depressed with inverted T wave in V_1 and V_2. T waves in leads I , V_5 and V_6 are upright.

[ECG Tracing] (Figure 4-29)

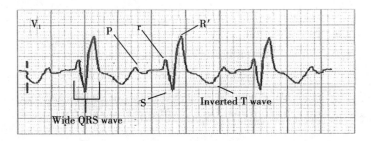

Figure 4-29   **Right bundle branch block.**

Left Bundle Branch Block

The sequence of depolarization changes into interventricular septum to the right ventricle to the left ventricle because of left bundle branch block. The end of QRS complex is prolonged with changed pattern (Figure 4-30).

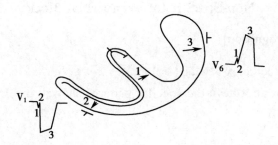

Figure 4-30   **The principle of changed pattern in QRS complex in LBBB.**

[ECG Recognition]

1. It is complete left bundle branch block when the duration of QRS complexes is greater than or equal to 0.12 s. Otherwise, it is incomplete left bundle branch block.
2. R wave is broad, with a round peak, or notched in leads I, aVL, V_5 and V_6.
3. Left axis deviation.
4. QRS complex resembles rS or QS configuration in leads V_1 and V_2. Q wave disappears in leads I, V_5 and V_6.
5. The duration of R wave is greater than 0.06 s in leads V_5 and V_6.
6. The direction of ST-T is opposite to that of QRS complex.

[ECG Tracing] (Figure 4-31)

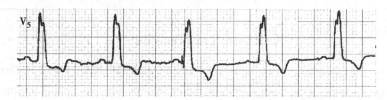

Figure 4-31　Left bundle branch block.

Non-Specific Intraventricular Block

[ECG Recognition]

1. QRS complex is wide ($\geqslant 0.12$ s).
2. It does not have the specific patterns showed in LBBB or RBBB.

[ECG Tracing] (Figure 4-32)

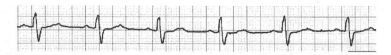

Figure 4-32   Non-specific intraventricular block.

Left Anterior Fascicular Block

[ECG Recognition]

1. A left axis deviation between $-30°$ and $-90°$ can be seen. An axis $\geqslant -45°$ is more suggestive of LAFB.

2. Leads II, III, and aVF show a rS pattern and the S wave in lead III is deeper than that in lead II. Lead aVL shows a qR pattern and the amplitude of the R wave in lead aVL is greater than that in lead I.

3. The duration of QRS complex is prolonged but is still less than 0.12 s.

[ECG Tracing] (Figure 4-33)

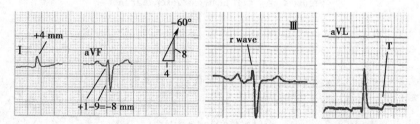

Figure 4-33   Left anterior fascicular block (hemiblock).

Left Posterior Fascicular Block

[ECG Recognition]

- A right axis deviation between +90° and +180°.
- Some rS patterns are seen in leads I and aVL, and qR patterns are seen in leads III and aVF. The duration of the Q wave is less than 0.025 s.
- The amplitude of the R wave is greater in lead III than that in lead II.
- The duration of QRS complex is less than 0.12 s.

[ECG Tracing] (Figure 4-34)

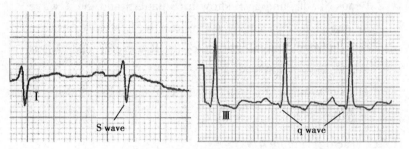

Figure 4-34   Left posterior fascicular block.

Wolff-Parkinson-White Syndrome (See Section 2 of Chapter 3)

Section 3   QRS Wave Absence

Ventricular Flutter

[ECG Recognition]

1. P wave is absent in all leads.
2. No identifiable QRS-T complex, but sine wave-like *flutter*

waves are shown.

3. Frequency: 200-250 bpm.

[ECG Tracing] (Figure 4-35)

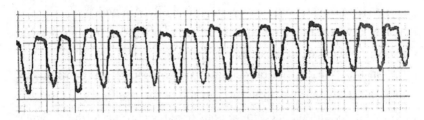

Figure 4-35   Ventricular flutter.

Ventricular Fibrillation

[ECG Recognition]

1. No visible QRS-T complex.
2. Rapid, coarse and irregular fibrillation waves are shown.
3. Frequency of fibrillation waves: 250 to 500 bpm.

[ECG Tracing] (Figure 4-36)

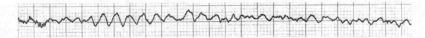

Figure 4-36   Ventricular fibrillation.

Section 4   Pathologic Q Waves

There are mainly two kinds of pathologic Q waves:

1. Q wave with abnormal morphology: the voltage (amplitude) of a normal Q wave is less than one fourth of that of the R wave in any given lead except lead aVR, and the duration of Q wave is less

than 0.04 s, or it should be defined as a pathologic Q wave

2. Abnormal presence of Q waves:

◆ Q or q wave is not supposed to be seen in lead V_1 or V_2 (but QS complex can be present in these leads).

◆ Q or q wave can be seen in leads aVR, aVL and Ⅲ.

◆ Q wave should not appear in leads Ⅰ, Ⅱ, aVF or V_4 to V_6 (but q wave can be seen in these leads).

In most cases, the presence of pathologic Q waves indicates transmural myocardial infarction in the corresponding site. But the following conditions need to be considered according to the patient's history:

◆ Myocarditis (Q wave is seen in leads V_1 to V_3).

◆ Hypertrophic cardiomyopathy (Q wave can be seen in leads Ⅱ, Ⅲ, aVF and V_4 to V_6).

◆ WPW syndrome (Q wave can be seen in leads Ⅱ, Ⅲ and aVF).

◆ Left ventricular hypertrophy (Q wave is seen in leads V_1 to V_3).

◆ LBBB (r wave is tiny or absent in leads Ⅱ, Ⅲ, aVF and V_1 to V_3).

◆ Massive pulmonary embolism (a Q wave is seen in leads V_1 to V_4).

Please find the pathologic Q wave in this strip (myocarditis, Figure 4-37).

History: 29-year-old male patient was healthy normally and had a cold one week before.

Please find the pathologic Q wave in this strip (hypertrophic cardiomyopathy, Figure 4-38).

History: 21-year-old female patient, diagnosed with hypertrophic cardiomyopathy confirmed by ultrasound.

Please find the pathologic Q wave in this strip (WPW syndrome, Figure 4-39).

History: the patient is a 40-year-old man whose medical reports showed some abnormalities in ECG.

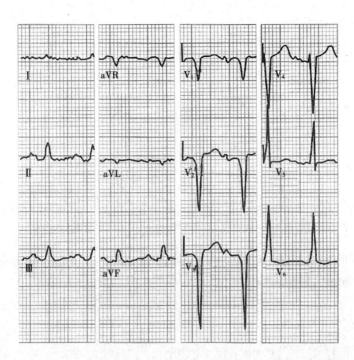

Figure 4-37   Pathologic Q wave in a patient with myocarditis.

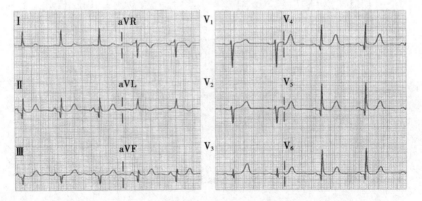

Figure 4-38   Pathologic Q wave in a patient with hypertrophic cardiomyopathy.

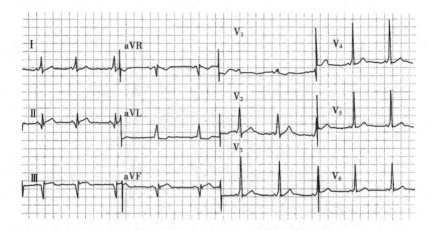

Figure 4-39   Pathologic Q wave in a patient with WPW syndrome.

Please find the pathologic Q wave in this strip (left ventricular hypertrophy, Figure 4-40).

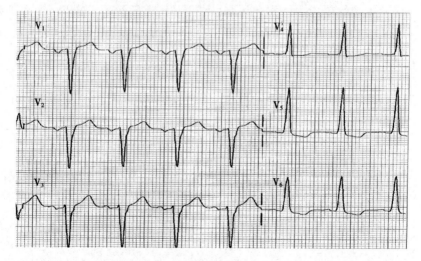

Figure 4-40   Pathologic Q wave in a patient with left ventricular hypertrophy.

History: 55-year-old male patient, diagnosed with dilated cardiomyopathy confirmed by ultrasound.

Please find the pathologic Q wave in this strip (LBBB, Figure 4-41).

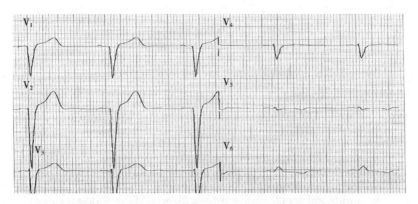

Figure 4-41   Pathologic Q wave in a patient with LBBB.

History: 19-year-old female patient. Abnormalities in ECG were discovered in a health check.

Please find the pathologic Q wave in this strip (massive pulmonary embolism, Figure 4-42).

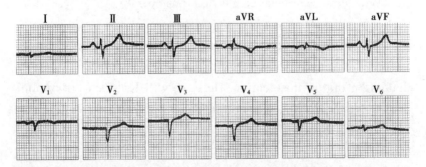

Figure 4-42   Pathologic Q wave in patient with massive pulmonary embolism.

History: 27-year-old female patient bedridden due to fractures. She complained of sudden chest pain and dyspnea.

Section 5　Common Type of Tachycardia with Wide QRS Complex

Wide QRS complex tachycardia refers to tachycardia with the duration of QRS complex ≥ 0.12 s and HR>100 bpm. The following types of wide QRS complex tachycardia are common in clinical practice:

1. Ventricular tachycardia (accounting for about 70% to 80% of wide QRS complex tachycardia).

2. Supraventricular tachycardia with any of the followings:

With aberrant intraventricular conduction (including bundle branch blocks or other types of intraventricular blocks, accounting for 15%).

With accessory pathway conduction (accounting for 1% to 5%).

With effect of medication or electrolyte disturbances.

With slow ventricular conduction (postoperative).

3. Ventricular pacing

Diagnosis of wide QRS complex SVT requires the ECG before the onset of tachycardia as reference, but we are not going into further details on this in this section. Here we will focus on differential diagnosis of VT versus wide QRS complex tachycardia.

Ventricular Tachycardia (VT)

[ECG Recognition]

1. Continuous wide QRS complexes, duration ≥ 0.12 s and HR>100 bpm.
2. Frequency: usually 150 to 200 bpm.
3. Tachycardia can be either paroxysmal or sustained.

4. If all QRS complexes have the same morphology and amplitude, the ECG variant is defined as monomorphic VT (Figure 4-43A). If 3 or more QRS complexes with distinct morphology appear in the same lead with a frequency of more than 200 bpm, and such pattern continues for ten or more heartbeats, the variant is defined as polymorphic VT (Figure 4-43B). Polymorphic VT can be subdivided into two types: sinus rhythm with normal Q-T intervals; sinus rhythm with prolonged Q-T intervals, which is usually torsade de pointes (Figure 4-43C).

[ECG tracing] (Figure 4-43)

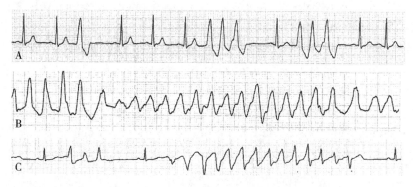

Figure 4-43   Ventricular tachycardia.
A: Monomorphic VT; B: Polymorphic VT; C: Torsades de pointes.

Differential Diagnosis of Wide QRS Complex Tachycardia

Ⅰ. Ventricular Rate and Ventricular Rhythm

Ventricular rate: In most VT cases, ventricular rate is between 150 and 200 bpm and ventricular rate of more than 180 bpm rarely happens. If this rate is too high, then it is more likely a SVT or atrial flutter with 1 ∶ 1 AV conduction rather than VT.

Ventricular rhythm: In VT, ventricular rhythm can be either regular or a bit irregular. However, in SVT the rhythm is strictly regular.

Ⅱ. Atrioventricular Dissociation (AV dissociation), Ventricular Capture and Ventricular Fusion Wave

If AV dissociation is present and ventricular rate is faster than atrial rate, the diagnosis of VT can be confirmed. In addition, ventricular capture and the appearance of ventricular fusion wave are important evidence for the diagnosis of VT.

Ⅲ. Duration of the QRS Complex

In general, the wider the QRS complex is, the greater possibility of VT is. A RBBB-like morphology with duration more than 0.14 s, or a LBBB-like morphology with duration more than 0.16 s is highly suggestive of VT. In a few cases, the duration of QRS complex in VT can be normal, such as in idiopathic ventricular tachycardia (IVT).

Ⅳ. Mean QRS Axis

If mean QRS axis lies between –90° and –180° (also known as extreme right axis deviation, northwest or no man's land), in most cases it's VT.

Ⅴ. QRS Complex in Chest Leads

◆ Concordant negative QRS complex pattern in chest leads indicates VT; concordant positive QRS complex pattern in chest leads, in most cases indicates VT and in a few cases is suggestive of atrioventricular reentry tachycardia (AVRT) involving a left accessory pathway.

◆ When tachycardia occurs, if QR, QS or qR pattern rather than RS pattern (including RS, rS and Rs complex) is present in leads V_1 to V_6, diagnosis of VT can be clearly confirmed. If RS pattern is present in leads V_1 to V_6 with duration of any RS waveform (the interval between the onset of R wave and the lowest point of S wave) more than 0.1 s, VT can also be confirmed (Figure 4-44).

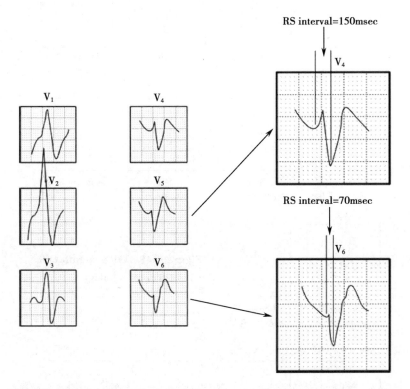

Figure 4-44   RS pattern in leads V₁ to V₆ and measuring duration of RS complex.

   ◆ Characteristics of QRS complex in leads V_1 and V_6: It is divided into RBBB-like morphology (positive mean electrical axes of QRS complexes in lead V_1, Figure 4-45) and LBBB-like morphology (negative mean electrical axes of QRS complexes in lead V_1, Figure 4-46).

   Ⅵ. A wide QRS complex tachycardia with LBBB morphology and obvious right axis deviation indicates the diagnosis of VT. Negative mean electrical axis in leads Ⅱ, Ⅲ and aVF is very likely to

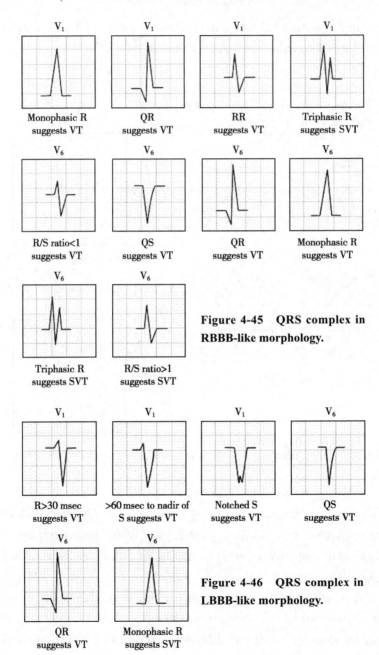

Figure 4-45 QRS complex in RBBB-like morphology.

Figure 4-46 QRS complex in LBBB-like morphology.

be an indication of VT.

Ⅶ. Precipitating Factors of Tachycardia

In most cases, tachycardia triggered by supraventricular premature contraction is SVT; tachycardia evoked by ventricular premature contraction is usually VT.

Ⅷ. Comparing ECG taken before onset of tachycardia: If the QRS complex is consistent in morphology with the complex in sinus rhythm, it usually indicates SVT; if not, it is likely to be VT.

According to clues above to diagnosis of VT, we can summarize the ECG recognition under the condition of definitive diagnosis of VT and probable VT, and hoped it could be helpful for clinical practice:

[You can make a definitive diagnosis of VT if:]

- The mean electrical axes of QRS complexes in leads V_1 to V_6 are negative.
- No RS pattern is in leads V_1 to V_6.
- RS pattern is present in leads V_1 to V_6, but RS duration is more than 0.1 s.
- Evident AV dissociation with ventricular rate greater than atrial rate.
- LBBB variant with right axis deviation.
- Concordant ECG tracing with ventricular premature contraction before the onset of tachycardia.
- Presence of tall positive R wave in lead aVR.

[VT highly probable if:]

- All the mean electrical axes of QRS complexes in leads V_1 to V_6 are positive.
- Severe right axis deviation.
- The duration of QRS complex is more than 0.16 s in LBBB-like morphology or more than 0.14 s in RBBB-like morphology.
- All the mean electrical axes of QRS complexes in leads Ⅱ, Ⅲ

and aVF are negative.

Section 6   ECG Practice Strips

Strip **4-1**   Rhythm (Regular   Irregular)   Rate (bpm)
P Wave (Sinus   Non-sinus   Absence)   P-R Interval (Prolonged/Shortened)
QRS Complex (Axis   Voltage   Widening   Absence of QRS Complex   Q Wave)

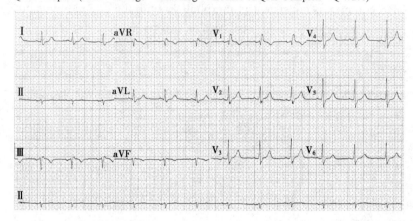

Strip **4-2**   Rhythm (Regular   Irregular)   Rate (bpm)
P Wave (Sinus   Non-sinus   Absence)   P-R Interval (Prolonged/Shortened)
QRS Complex (Axis   Voltage   Widening   Absence of QRS Complex   Q Wave)

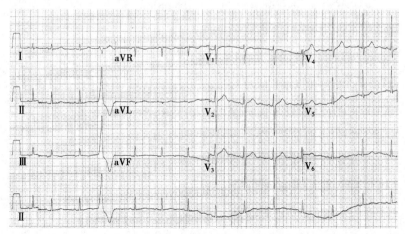

Strip **4-3**   Rhythm (Regular   Irregular)   Rate (bpm)
P Wave (Sinus   Non-sinus   Absence)   P-R Interval (Prolonged/Shortened)
QRS Complex (Axis   Voltage   Widening   Absence of QRS Complex   Q Wave)

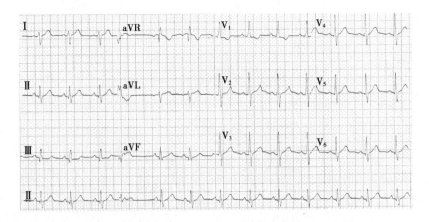

Strip **4-4**   Rhythm (Regular   Irregular)   Rate (bpm)
P Wave (Sinus   Non-sinus   Absence)   P-R Interval (Prolonged/Shortened)
QRS Complex (Axis   Voltage   Widening   Absence of QRS Complex   Q Wave)

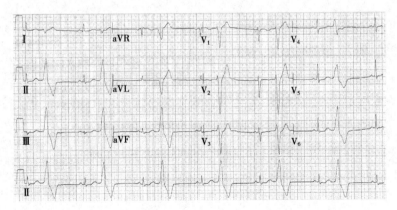

Strip **4-5**   Rhythm (Regular   Irregular)   Rate (bpm)

P Wave (Sinus   Non-sinus   Absence)   P-R Interval (Prolonged/Shortened)

QRS Complex (Axis   Voltage   Widening   Absence of QRS Complex   Q Wave)

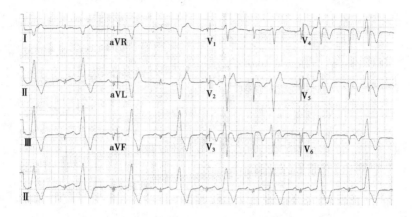

Strip **4-6**   Rhythm (Regular   Irregular)   Rate (bpm)

P Wave (Sinus   Non-sinus   Absence)   P-R Interval (Prolonged/Shortened)

QRS Complex (Axis   Voltage   Widening   Absence of QRS Complex   Q Wave)

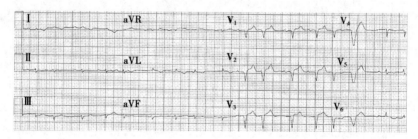

Strip **4-7**　Rhythm (Regular　Irregular)　Rate (　　bpm)
P Wave (Sinus　Non-sinus　Absence)　P-R Interval (Prolonged/Shortened)
QRS Complex (Axis　Voltage　Widening　Absence of QRS Complex　Q Wave)

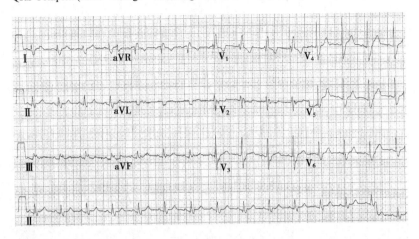

Strip **4-8**　Rhythm (Regular　Irregular)　Rate (　　bpm)
P Wave (Sinus　Non-sinus　Absence)　P-R Interval (Prolonged/Shortened)
QRS Complex (Axis　Voltage　Widening　Absence of QRS Complex　Q Wave)

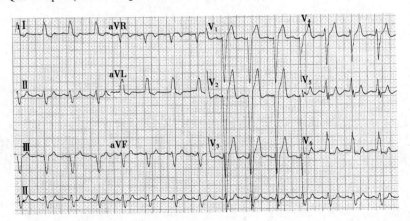

Strip **4-9** Rhythm (Regular   Irregular)   Rate (bpm)
P Wave (Sinus   Non-sinus   Absence)   P-R Interval (Prolonged/Shortened)
QRS Complex (Axis   Voltage   Widening   Absence of QRS Complex   Q Wave)

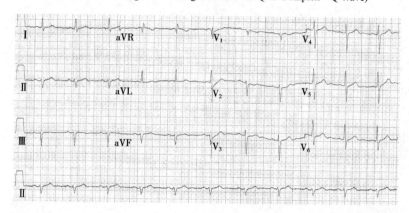

Strip **4-10** Rhythm (Regular   Irregular)   Rate (bpm)
P Wave (Sinus   Non-sinus   Absence)   P-R Interval (Prolonged/Shortened)
QRS Complex (Axis   Voltage   Widening   Absence of QRS Complex   Q Wave)

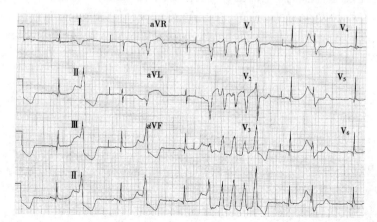

Strip **4-11**   Rhythm (Regular   Irregular)   Rate (bpm)
P Wave (Sinus   Non-sinus   Absence)   P-R Interval (Prolonged/Shortened)
QRS Complex (Axis   Voltage   Widening   Absence of QRS Complex   Q Wave)

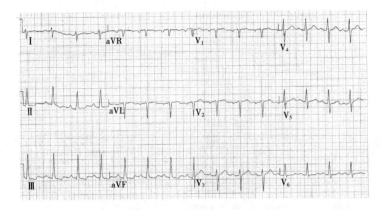

Strip **4-12**   Rhythm (Regular   Irregular)   Rate (bpm)
P Wave (Sinus   Non-sinus   Absence)   P-R Interval (Prolonged/Shortened)
QRS Complex (Axis   Voltage   Widening   Absence of QRS Complex   Q Wave)

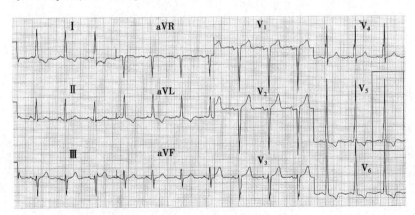

Strip **4-13** Rhythm (Regular Irregular) Rate (bpm)
P Wave (Sinus Non-sinus Absence) P-R Interval (Prolonged/Shortened)
QRS Complex (Axis Voltage Widening Absence of QRS Complex Q Wave)

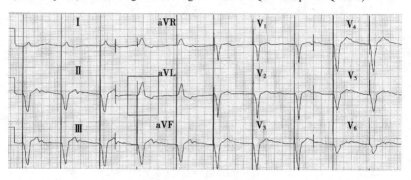

Strip **4-14** Rhythm (Regular Irregular) Rate (bpm)
P wave (Sinus Non-sinus Absence) P-R Interval (Prolonged/Shortened)
QRS complex (Axis Voltage Widening Absence of QRS Complex Q wave)

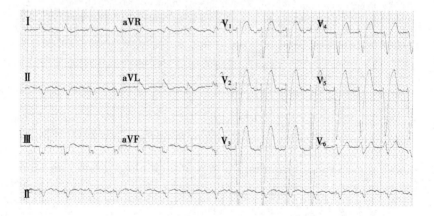

Strip **4-15**　Rhythm (Regular　Irregular)　Rate (　　bpm)

P Wave (Sinus　Non-sinus　Absence)　P-R Interval (Prolonged/Shortened)

QRS Complex (Axis　Voltage　Widening　Absence of QRS Complex　Q Wave)

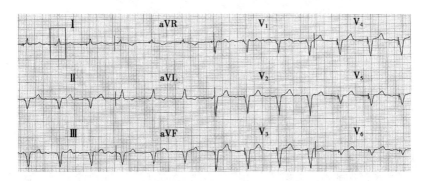

Strip **4-16**　Rhythm (Regular　Irregular)　Rate (　　bpm)

P Wave (Sinus　Non-sinus　Absence)　P-R Interval (Prolonged/Shortened)

QRS Complex (Axis　Voltage　Widening　Absence of QRS Complex　Q Wave)

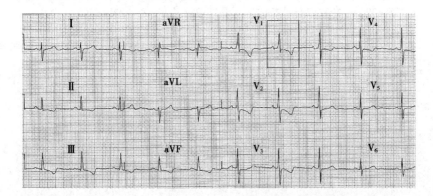

Strip **4-17** Rhythm (Regular   Irregular)   Rate (bpm)
P Wave (Sinus   Non-sinus   Absence)   P-R Interval (Prolonged/Shortened)
QRS Complex (Axis   Voltage   Widening   Absence of QRS Complex   Q Wave)

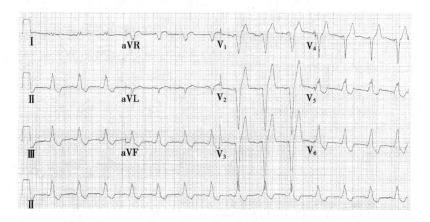

Strip **4-18** Rhythm (Regular   Irregular)   Rate (bpm)
P Wave (Sinus   Non-sinus   Absence)   P-R Interval (Prolonged/Shortened)
QRS Complex (Axis   Voltage   Widening   Absence of QRS Complex   Q Wave)

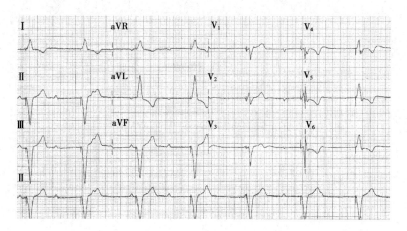

Strip **4-19**   Rhythm (Regular   Irregular)   Rate (bpm)

P Wave (Sinus   Non-sinus   Absence)   P-R Interval (Prolonged/Shortened)

QRS Complex (Axis   Voltage   Widening   Absence of QRS Complex   Q Wave)

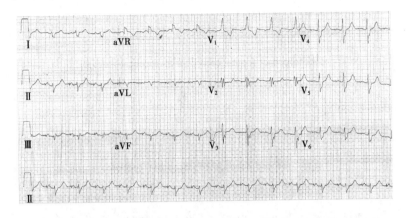

Strip **4-20**   Rhythm (Regular   Irregular)   Rate (bpm)

P Wave (Sinus   Non-sinus   Absence)   P-R Interval (Prolonged/Shortened)

QRS Complex (Axis   Voltage   Widening   Absence of QRS Complex   Q Wave)

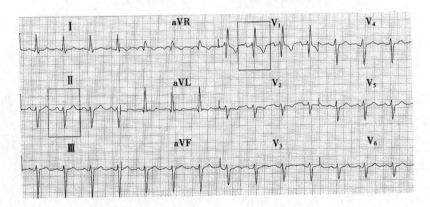

Strip **4-21**　Rhythm (Regular　Irregular)　Rate (　　bpm)
P Wave (Sinus　Non-sinus　Absence)　P-R Interval (Prolonged/Shortened)
QRS Complex (Axis　Voltage　Widening　Absence of QRS Complex　Q Wave)

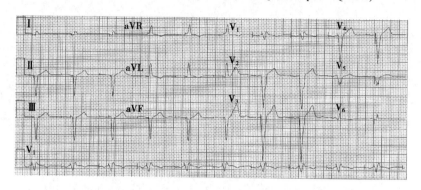

Strip **4-22**　Rhythm (Regular　Irregular)　Rate (　　bpm)
P Wave (Sinus　Non-sinus　Absence)　P-R Interval (Prolonged/Shortened)
QRS Complex (Axis　Voltage　Widening　Absence of QRS Complex　Q Wave)

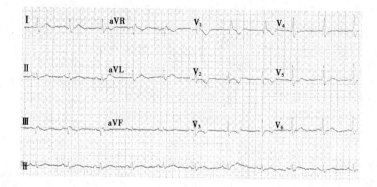

Strip **4-23**   Rhythm (Regular   Irregular)   Rate (bpm)
P Wave (Sinus   Non-sinus   Absence)   P-R Interval (Prolonged/Shortened)
QRS Complex (Axis   Voltage   Widening   Absence of QRS Complex   Q Wave)

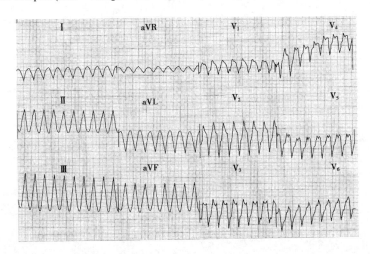

Strip **4-24**   Rhythm (Regular   Irregular)   Rate (bpm)
P Wave (Sinus   Non-sinus   Absence)   P-R Interval (Prolonged/Shortened)
QRS Complex (Axis   Voltage   Widening   Absence of QRS Complex   Q Wave)

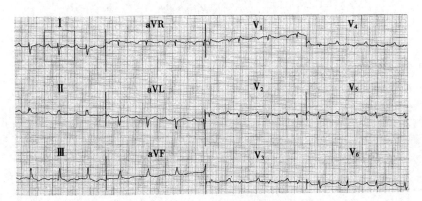

Strip **4-25** Rhythm (Regular Irregular) Rate (bpm)
P Wave (Sinus Non-sinus Absence) P-R Interval (Prolonged/Shortened)
QRS Complex (Axis Voltage Widening Absence of QRS Complex Q Wave)

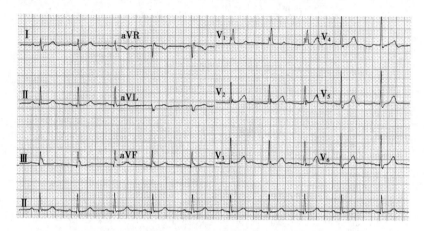

Strip **4-26** Rhythm (Regular Irregular) Rate (bpm)
P Wave (Sinus Non-sinus Absence) P-R Interval (Prolonged/Shortened)
QRS Complex (Axis Voltage Widening Absence of QRS Complex Q Wave)

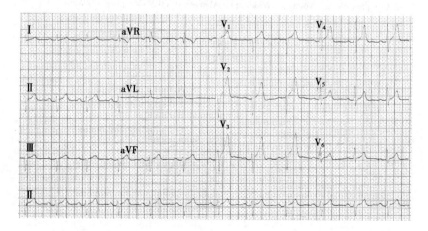

Answers to the Strips

Strip 4-1　Rhythm: Regular　Rate: 60 to 100 bpm
P wave: Sinus P wave　P-R Interval: Normal
QRS Complex: Left axis deviation, rS pattern in leads
II, III, and aVF, qR pattern in lead aVL. 'M'-shaped
premature QRS complex in lead V_1
Diagnosis: Sinus rhythm, left anterior fascicular block,
complete right bundle block

Strip 4-2　Rhythm: Irregular　Rate: 60 to 100 bpm
P Wave: Sinus P wave　P-R Interval: Normal
QRS Complex: Normal axis, premature wide QRS wave
Diagnosis: Sinus rhythm, premature ventricular contraction

Strip 4-3　Rhythm: Regular　Rate: 60 to 100 bpm
P Wave: Sinus P wave　P-R Interval: Normal
QRS Complex: Right axis deviation, tall R wave in lead
V_1, premature wide QRS wave
Diagnosis: Sinus rhythm, high voltage in right ventricular
leads (right ventricular hypertrophy), premature ventricular
contraction

Strip 4-4　Rhythm: Regular　Rate: 60 to 100 bpm
P Wave: Sinus P wave　P-R Interval: Normal
QRS Complex: Normal axis, normal voltage, premature
wide QRS complex
Diagnosis: Sinus rhythm, premature ventricular contraction
(bigeminy)

Strip 4-5   Rhythm: Regular   Rate: 60 to 100 bpm
P Wave: Sinus P wave   P-R Interval: Normal
QRS Complex: Normal axis, normal voltage, premature wide QRS complex
Diagnosis: Sinus rhythm, premature ventricular contraction (bigeminy)

Strip 4-6   Rhythm: Regular   Rate: more than 100 bpm
P Wave: Sinus P wave   P-R Interval: Normal
QRS Complex: Normal axis, low voltage in whole QRS complex
Diagnosis: Sinus tachycardia, low voltage in whole leads (both chest leads and limb leads)

Strip 4-7   Rhythm: Regular   Rate: 60 to 100 bpm
P Wave: Sinus P wave   P-R Interval: Normal
QRS Complex: Normal axis, 'M'-shaped premature QRS complex in lead V_1
Diagnosis: Sinus rhythm, complete right bundle block

Strip 4-8   Rhythm: Regular   Rate: 60 to 100 bpm
P Wave: Sinus P wave   P-R Interval: Normal
QRS Complex: Left axis deviation, 'M'-shaped premature QRS complex in leads I、aVL、V_5 and V_6
Diagnosis: Sinus rhythm, complete left bundle branch block

Strip 4-9   Rhythm: Regular   Rate: 60 to 100 bpm
P Wave: Sinus P wave   P-R Interval: Normal
QRS Complex: Left axis deviation, rS pattern in leads II,

Ⅲ, and aVF, qR pattern in lead aVL

Diagnosis: Sinus rhythm, left anterior fascicular block

Strip 4-10   Rhythm: Irregular   Rate: 60 to 100 bpm
P Wave: Sinus P wave   P-R Interval: Normal
QRS Complex: Normal axis, premature wide QRS complex, sometimes more than 3 complexes
Diagnosis: Sinus rhythm, premature ventricular contraction, paroxysmal supraventricular tachycardia

Strip 4-11   Rhythm: Regular   Rate: 60 to 100 bpm
P Wave: Sinus P wave   P-R Interval: Normal
QRS Complex: Right axis deviation, rS pattern in leads Ⅰ and aVL, qR in lead aVF
Diagnosis: Sinus rhythm, left posterior fascicular block

Strip 4-12   Rhythm: Regular   Rate: 60 to 100 bpm
P Wave: Sinus P wave   P-R Interval: Normal
QRS Complex: Normal axis, apparent voltage abnormality
Diagnosis: Sinus rhythm, high voltage in left ventricular leads (left ventricular hypertrophy)

Strip 4-13   Rhythm: Regular   Rate: approximately 60 bpm
P Wave: Absence of sinus P wave
QRS Complex: Wide QRS complex, apparent pacemaker spike at the start of the QRS complex
Diagnosis: Paced ECG (unipolar pacing in VVI)

Strip 4-14   Rhythm: Regular   Rate: 60 to 100 bpm
P wave: Sinus P wave   P-R Interval: Normal

QRS Complex: Unapparent left deviation, apparent voltage abnormality, 'M'-shaped QRS complex in leads Ⅰ, aVL, V_5, V_6

Diagnosis: Sinus rhythm, high voltage in left ventricular leads, complete left bundle branch block

Strip 4-15   Rhythm: Regular   Rate: 60 to 100 bpm

P wave: absence of sinus P wave

QRS Complex: Wide QRS complex, apparent pacemaker spike at the start of the QRS complex

Diagnosis: Atrial fibrillation, paced ECG (bipolar pacing in VVI)

Strip 4-16   Rhythm: Regular   Rate: more than 100 bpm

P wave: Sinus P wave   P-R Interval: Apparently shortened P-R interval

QRS Complex: Right axis deviation, tall R wave in lead V_1, wide QRS complex with delta wave at its beginning

Diagnosis: Sinus tachycardia, high voltage in right ventricular leads (right ventricular hypertrophy), WPW syndrome

Strip 4-17   Rhythm: Regular   Rate: 60 to 100 bpm

P wave: absence of sinus P wave (apparent pacemaker spike at the start)

QRS Complex: Wide QRS complex, apparent pacemaker spike at the start of the QRS complex

Diagnosis: Paced ECG (bipolar pacing in DDD)

Strip 4-18   Rhythm: Regular   Rate: 60 to 100 bpm

P wave: Sinus P wave (absence of relevant QRS complex afterwards)

QRS Complex: Wide QRS complex, apparent pacemaker spike at the start of the QRS complex

Diagnosis: 3rd degree heart block, paced ECG (bipolar pacing in VVI)

Strip 4-19 Rhythm: Regular　Rate: 60 to 100 bpm

P wave: Non-sinus P wave (apparent pacemaker spike at the start)

QRS Complex: Normal axis, voltage, and QRS duration

Diagnosis: Paced ECG (bipolar pacing in AAI)

Strip 4-20 Rhythm: Regular　Rate: 60 to 100 bpm

P wave: sinus P wave　P-R Interval: Normal

QRS complex: Left axis deviation, rS pattern in leads II, III, aVF, qR pattern in leads I, aVL, 'M'-shaped QRS in lead V_1

Diagnosis: Sinus tachycardia, left anterior fascicular block, complete right bundle block

Strip 4-21 Rhythm: Regular　Rate: 60 to 100 bpm

P wave: Absence of sinus P wave (apparent pacemaker spike before P wave)

QRS Complex: Wide QRS complex, apparent pacemaker spike at the start of the QRS complex

Diagnosis: Paced ECG (bipolar pacing in DDD)

Strip 4-22 Rhythm: Regular　Rate: 60 to 100 bpm

P wave: sinus P wave　P-R Interval: Normal

QRS Complex: Normal axis, 'M'-shaped QRS complex in lead V_1

Diagnosis: Sinus rhythm, complete right bundle block

Strip 4-23　Rhythm: Regular　Rate: More than 100 bpm

P wave: Non-sinus P wave

QRS Complex: Tachycardia with wide QRS complex (no RS pattern in chest leads)

Diagnosis: Ventricular tachycardia

Strip 4-24　Rhythm: Regular　Rate: 60 to 100 bpm

P wave: Sinus P wave　　P-R Interval: Normal

QRS Complex: Right axis deviation, rS pattern in leads I and aVL, qR pattern in leads II, III, aVF

Diagnosis: Sinus rhythm, left posterior fascicular block

Strip 4-25　Rhythm: Regular　Rate: 60 to 100 bpm

P wave: Sinus P wave　P-R Interval: Normal

QRS Complex: Normal axis, 'M'-shaped QRS in lead V_1

Diagnosis: Sinus rhythm, complete right bundle block

Strip 4-26　Rhythm: Regular　Rate: 60 to 100 bpm

P wave: Sinus P wave　P-R Interval: Normal

QRS Complex: Left axis deviation, rS pattern in leads II, III and aVF, qR pattern in leads I and aVL

Diagnosis: Sinus rhythm, left anterior fascicular block

Chapter 5

ST Segment

ST segment refers to the line connecting the end of QRS complex and the beginning of T wave. Pathologically, ECG tracing may show ST segment elongation or shortening, but more often the elevation and depression, such as the ST pattern in myocardium ischemia (MI). So in MI, as the ST vector points from normal myocardial cells to abnormal ones, ST segment elevation could be seen on patients with subepicardial ischemia (transmural myocardial ischemia), and the direction of vector is from endocardium to epicardium and ST segment depression on those with subendocardial ischemia, with the direction of vector from epicardium to endocardium. Besides, it is worth noting that MI can generally disturb the normal depolarization of ventricular myocardium, which may lead to some other ST abnormal signs on ECG tracing.

However, these changes are not specific for MI, and they could also be attributed to organic cardiac disease, electrolyte disturbances or effect of drugs. It is even seen on some normal people. Therefore, it's important to consider clinical symptoms when analyzing ECG tracing and be cautious to dynamic changes.

Section 1   Normal ST Segment

[ECG Recognition]

1. ST segment at baseline without deviation.

2. Deviation within normal range:

Depression of ST segment less than **0.05 mV** in all leads.

Elevation less than 0.1 mV in all limb leads and leads V_4 to V_6, less than 0.3 mV in leads V_1 and V_2, less than 0.5 mV in lead V_3.

Section 2   Abnormal ST Segment

I. ST Segment Elevation

ST segment elevation can be caused by many reasons, among which acute myocardial infarction (AMI), early repolarization syndrome, acute pericarditis, ventricular hypertrophy (more details in Chapter 4.2) and bundle branch block (more details on Chapter 4.2) are more common.

Acute Myocardial Infarction

AMI is a severe and common cardiac disease showing as ST elevated myocardial infaction. And the ECG tracing of such patients can be very regular, thus providing meaningful ECG proof for clinical physicians. We could also divide AMI into phases by their ECG tracings (Figure 5-1 to Figure 5-4). However, these phases are defined artificially, and these typical changes do not appear on everyone. One should always consider individual variation and be flexible about interpretation of the tracing. Typical ECG changes of AMI are as follows:

Superacute Phase (early phase, minutes to hours)

[ECG Recognition] (Figure 5-1)

1. Tall, upright and symmetrical T wave.
2. ST elevation with obliquely straight morphology.
3. No pathological Q wave.

[ECG Tracing] (Figure 5-1)

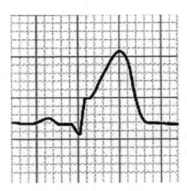

Figure 5-1　ST segment changes in superacute phase.

Acute Phase (hours/days to weeks)

[ECG Recognition]

1. Inverted T wave.
2. ST elevation with obliquely straight morphology/convex.
3. Pathological Q wave.

[ECG Tracing] (Figure 5-2)

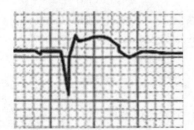

Figure 5-2　ST segment changes in acute phase.

Subacute Phase (weeks to months)

[ECG Recognition]

1. Inverted T waves but smaller, ST segment at baseline.
2. Pathological Q wave.

[ECG Tracing] (Figure 5-3)

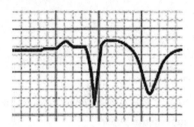

Figure 5-3　ST segment changes in subacute phase.

Recovery Phase (several months later)

[ECG Recognition]

1. T wave upright without changes anymore.
2. ST segment at baseline without more change.
3. Pathological Q wave.

[ECG Tracing] (Figure 5-4)

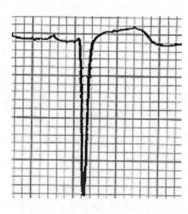

Figure 5-4　ST segment changes in recovery phase.

Besides, the ECG can tell the location of myocardial infarction based on the leads in which the basic patterns of myocardial infarction present.

1. Inferior wall: leads Ⅱ, Ⅲ, aVF.

2. Anterior wall: leads V_1, V_2, V_3, V_4, V_5, V_6.

3. Lateral wall: leads V_5, V_6, Ⅰ, aVL.

4. Posterior wall: leads V_7, V_8, V_9, V_1, V_2 with R waves and peaked T waves.

5. Right ventricle: leads V_3R, V_4R, V_5R, V_6R.

The hexaxial reference system and axes of the chest leads may help us memorize the location of myocardial infarction (Figure 5-5).

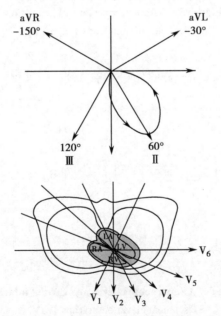

Figure 5-5   The hexaxial reference system and the axes of chest leads.

Using what you learned above, analyze the following practice strips and find out the location and phase of myocardial infarction (Figure 5-6 to Figure 5-9).

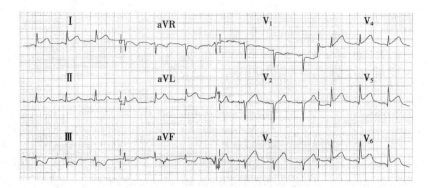

Figure 5-6   Acute anterolateral infarction.

ST segment elevation in leads I, aVL, V$_2$ to V$_6$.

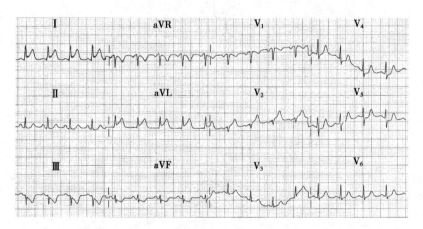

Figure 5-7   Superacute lateral myocardial infarction.

ST segment elevation in leads I, aVL.

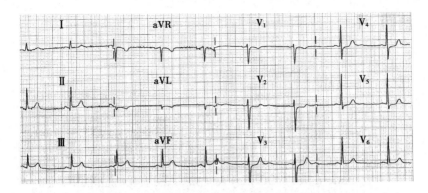

Figure 5-8 Superacute inferior myocardial infarction.

ST segment elevation in leads II, III, aVF, tall and peaked T wave.

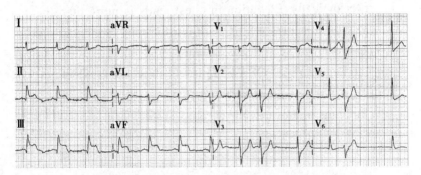

Figure 5-9 Acute inferior myocardial infarction.

ST segment elevation in leads II, III, aVF.

Early Repolarization Syndrome

Early repolarization syndrome is a common disease in clinical settings that can be revealed by ECG. It refers to a 0.1 mV elevation of J point (the border of the ending of QRS complex and the beginning of ST segment in at least two neighboring leads).

Two common types of ECG variant can be discovered in early depolarization syndrome: smooth transition from QRS complex to the ST segment instead of a sharp turn, called J point; the other for a deflection or upright wavelet between QRS complex and ST segment, called J wave (Figure 5-10).

[ECG Recognition]

1. J point elevation and J wave formation: mainly in leads V_2 to V_5, occasionally seen in leads II, III, aVF. When the J wave is present in leads V_1, V_2 and QRS complex changes to rSr' pattern, the ECG may resemble the right bundle branch block variant.

2. Concave ST elevation is commonly seen in chest leads and inferior leads. Elevation in chest leads is more than that in inferior leads, usually within a 0.5 mV gap. A tall and peaked T wave could also present.

3. The beginning of QRS complex is slow but the declining part is fast, or with a notch or deflection. The QRS complex's amplitude improves while duration is shortened.

[ECG Tracing] (Figure 5-10)

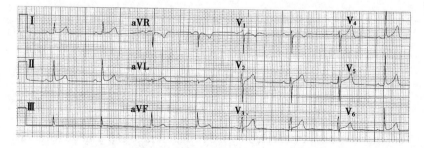

Figure 5-10   Early repolarization syndrome.

Acute Pericarditis

Acute pericarditis is an acute inflammation of the pericardium, both visceral and parietal layer. It might occur with myocarditis and endocarditis or as the only cardiac impairment. ECG of patients with acute pericarditis is dynamic, as shown in Figure 5-11.

[ECG Recognition]

1. Sinus rhythm: normal rate or sinus bradycardia, sinus tachycardia could also be seen.
2. P-R segment deviation: from 0.05 mV to 0.15mV (taking TP segment as the baseline).
3. Concave ST segment elevation and tall T wave: P-R segment deviation and ST segment elevation usually happen within several days to two weeks.
4. ST segment returns to baseline and T wave becomes flat gradually.
5. Inverted T wave is present and grows to the deepest (in lead aVR it could be upright) and usually maintains for several weeks, months or longer.
6. T wave returns upright, usually within three months.

[ECG Tracing] (Figure 5-11)

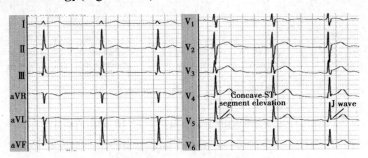

Figure 5-11   Acute pericarditis.

II. ST Segment Depression

Many diseases can cause ST segment depression, such as myocardial ischemia (Figure 5-12 to Figure 5-14), ventricular hypertrophy (more details in Chapter 4.2) and bundle branch block (more details in Chapter 4.2).

Myocardial Ischemia

[ECG Recognition]

> 1. P-R segment is usually used as the baseline to compare and judge the ST segment depression.
> 2. ST segment depression are various (more details on Chapter one), such as J point depression, up-sloping depression, horizontal depression and down-sloping depression, the specificity for ST segment to diagnosis of myocardial ischemia improves gradually (Figure 5-12).

[ECG Tracing] (Figure 5-12)

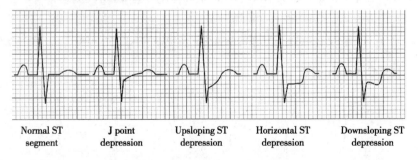

| Normal ST segment | J point depression | Upsloping ST depression | Horizontal ST depression | Downsloping ST depression |

Figure 5-12　Myocardial ischemia.

Please using what you learned above to analyze the following practice strips and find out the location of myocardial infarction (Figure 5-13, Figure 5-14):

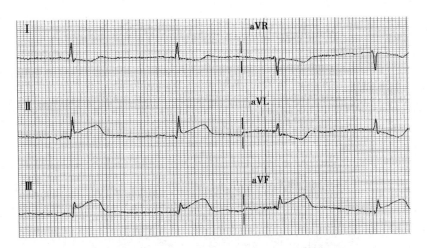

Figure 5-13   Acute inferior myocardial infarction.

ST segment elevation in leads Ⅱ, Ⅲ, aVF.

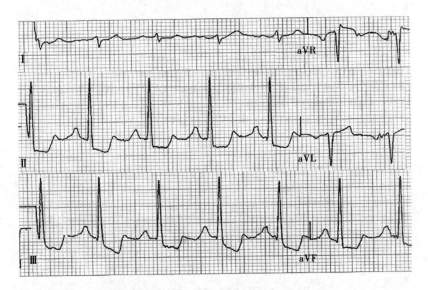

Figure 5-14   Inferior myocardial ischemia.

ST segment depression in leads Ⅱ, Ⅲ, aVF.

Section 3 ECG Practice Strips

Strip **5-1** Rhythm (Regular Irregular) Rate (bpm)
P Wave (Sinus Non-sinus Absent) P-R Interval (Prolonged/Shortened)
QRS Complex (Axis Voltage Widening Absence of QRS Complex Q Wave)
ST Segment (Elevated/ Depressed)
ST Segment Change in Leads (I , II , III , aVR, aVL, aVF, V$_1$, V$_2$, V$_3$, V$_4$, V$_5$, V$_6$).

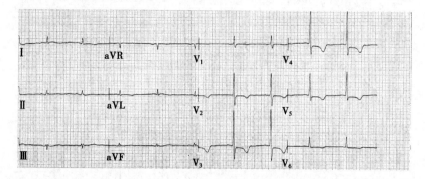

Strip **5-2** Rhythm (Regular Irregular) Rate (bpm)
P Wave (Sinus Non-sinus Absent) P-R Interval (Prolonged/Shortened)
QRS Complex (Axis Voltage Widening Absence of QRS Complex Q Wave)
ST Segment (Elevated/ Depressed)
ST Segment Change in Leads (I , II , III , aVR, aVL, aVF,V$_1$,V$_2$,V$_3$,V$_4$, V$_5$, V$_6$)

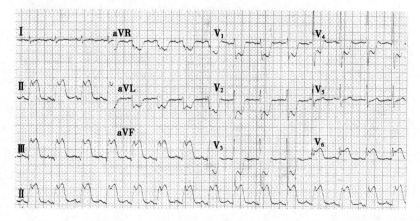

Strip **5-3**   Rhythm (Regular   Irregular)   Rate (bpm)

P Wave (Sinus   Non-sinus   Absent)   P-R Interval (Prolonged/Shortened)

QRS Complex (Axis   Voltage   Widening   Absence of QRS Complex   Q Wave)

ST Segment (Elevated/ Depressed)

ST Segment Change in Leads (I , II , III, aVR, aVL, aVF, V_1, V_2, V_3, V_4, V_5, V_6)

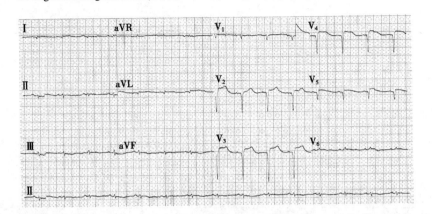

Strip **5-4**   Rhythm (Regular   Irregular)   Rate (bpm)

P Wave (Sinus   Non-sinus   Absent)   P-R Interval (Prolonged/Shortened)

QRS Complex (Axis   Voltage   Widening   Absence of QRS Complex   Q Wave)

ST Segment (Elevated/ Depressed)

ST Segment Change in Leads (I , II , III, aVR, aVL, aVF, V_1, V_2, V_3, V_4, V_5, V_6)

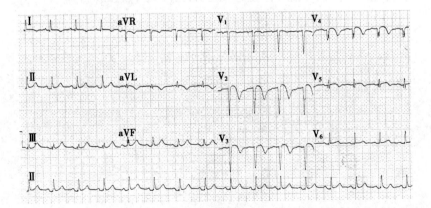

Strip **5-5** Rhythm (Regular Irregular) Rate (bpm)

P Wave (Sinus Non-sinus Absent) P-R Interval (Prolonged/Shortened)

QRS Complex (Axis Voltage Widening Absence of QRS Complex Q Wave)

ST Segment (Elevated/ Depressed)

ST Segment Change in Leads (I , II , III , aVR, aVL, aVF, V_1, V_2,V_3,V_4,V_5, V_6)

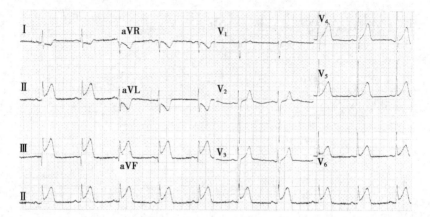

Strip **5-6** Rhythm (Regular Irregular) Rate (bpm)

P Wave (Sinus Non-sinus Absent) P-R Interval (Prolonged/Shortened)

QRS Complex (Axis Voltage Widening Absence of QRS Complex Q Wave)

ST Segment (Elevated/ Depressed)

ST Segment Change in Leads (I , II , III , aVR, aVL, aVF, V_1, V_2,V_3,V_4,V_5, V_6)

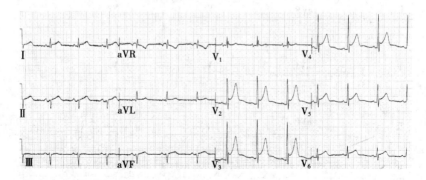

Strip **5-7**   Rhythm (Regular   Irregular)   Rate (bpm)

P Wave (Sinus   Non-sinus   Absent)   P-R Interval (Prolonged/Shortened)

QRS Complex (Axis   Voltage   Widening   Absence of QRS Complex   Q Wave)

ST Segment (Elevated/ Depressed)

ST Segment Change in Leads(I , II , III, aVR, aVL, aVF, V₁, V₂,V₃,V₄,V₅, V₆)

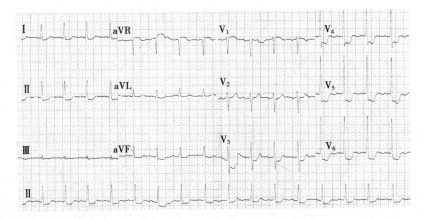

Strip **5-8**   Rhythm (Regular   Irregular)   Rate (bpm)

P Wave (Sinus   Non-sinus   Absent)   P-R Interval (Prolonged/Shortened)

QRS Complex (Axis   Voltage   Widening   Absence of QRS Complex   Q Wave)

ST Segment (Elevated/ Depressed)

ST Segment Change in Leads(I , II , III, aVR, aVL, aVF, V₁, V₂, V₃, V₄,V₅, V₆)

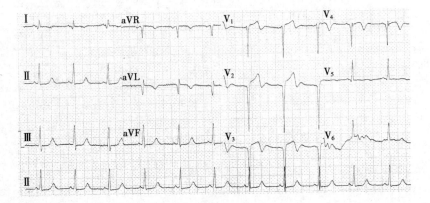

Strip **5-9** Rhythm (Regular　Irregular)　Rate (　　bpm)

P Wave (Sinus　Non-sinus　Absent)　P-R Interval (Prolonged/Shortened)

QRS Complex (Axis　Voltage　Widening　Absence of QRS Complex　Q Wave)

ST Segment (Elevated/ Depressed)

ST Segment Change in Leads(I , II , III, aVR, aVL, aVF, V_1, V_2, V_3, V_4, V_5, V_6)

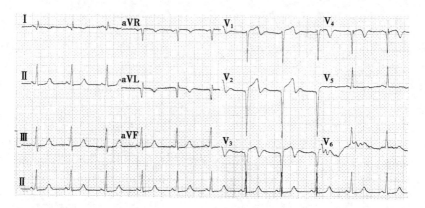

Strip **5-10** Rhythm (Regular　Irregular)　Rate (　　bpm)

P Wave (Sinus　Non-sinus　Absent)　P-R Interval (Prolonged/Shortened)

QRS Complex (Axis　Voltage　Widening　Absence of QRS Complex　Q Wave)

ST Segment (Elevated/ Depressed)

ST Segment Change in Leads (I , II , III, aVR, aVL, aVF, V_1, V_2, V_3, V_4, V_5, V_6)

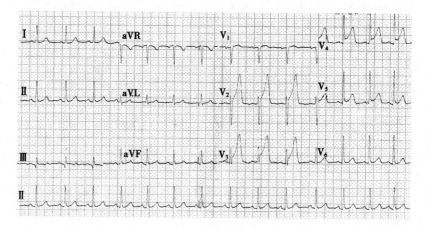

Strip **5-11** Rhythm (Regular Irregular) Rate (bpm)

P Wave (Sinus Non-sinus Absent) P-R Interval (Prolonged/Shortened)

QRS Complex (Axis Voltage Widening Absence of QRS Complex Q Wave)

ST Segment (Elevated/ Depressed)

ST Segment Change in Leads (I , II , III , aVR, aVL, aVF, V₁, V₂, V₃, V₄, V₅, V₆)

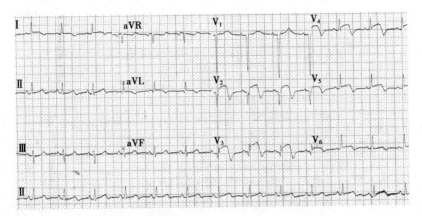

Strip **5-12** Rhythm (Regular Irregular) Rate (bpm)

P Wave (Sinus Non-sinus Absent) P-R Interval (Prolonged/Shortened)

QRS Complex (Axis Voltage Widening Absence of QRS Complex Q Wave)

ST Segment (Elevated/ Depressed)

ST Segment Change in Leads (I , II , III , aVR, aVL, aVF, V₁, V₂, V₃, V₄, V₅, V₆)

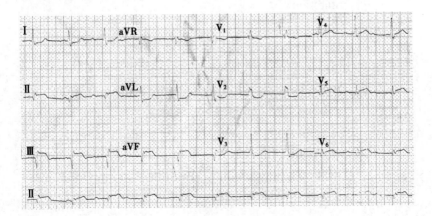

Answers to the Strips

Strip 5-1   Rhythm: Regular   Rate: 60-100 bpm

P Wave: Sinus   P-R Interval: Normal

QRS Complex: No axis deviation, low voltage in limb leads, abnormal voltage in chest leads

ST Segment: ST segment depression in leads V_3 to V_6

Diagnosis: Sinus rhythm, low voltage in limb leads, high voltage in left and right ventricles (biventricular hypertrophy), ST segment change (caused by ventricular hypertrophy, a sign of myocardial strain)

Strip 5-2   Rhythm: Regular   Rate: 60-100 bpm

P Wave: Sinus   P-R Interval: Normal

QRS Complex: No axis deviation, normal voltage, no QRS complex broadening

ST Segment: ST segment elevation in leads II, III, aVF; ST segment depression in leads V_1 to V_4

Diagnosis: Sinus rhythm, superacute inferior myocardial infarction

Strip 5-3   Rhythm: Regular   Rate: 60-100 bpm

P Wave: Sinus   P-R Interval: Normal

QRS Complex: No axis deviation, low voltage in limb leads, no QRS complex broadening

ST Segment: ST segment elevation in leads V_1 to V_4, pathologic Q wave

Diagnosis: Sinus rhythm, low voltage in limb leads, acute anterior myocardial infarction

Strip 5-4   Rhythm: Regular   Rate: 60-100 bpm
P Wave: Sinus   P-R Interval: Normal
QRS Complex: No axis deviation, normal voltage, no
QRS complex broadening
ST Segment: Convex ST elevation in leads V_1 to V_5,
pathologic Q wave
Diagnosis: Sinus rhythm, acute anterior myocardial
infarction

Strip 5-5   Rhythm: Regular   Rate: 60-100 bpm
P Wave: Sinus   P-R Interval: Normal
QRS Complex: No axis deviation, normal voltage, no
QRS complex broadening
ST Segment: ST segment elevation in leads Ⅱ, Ⅲ, aVF
Diagnosis: Sinus rhythm, superacute inferior myocardial
infarction

Strip 5-6   Rhythm: Regular   Rate: 60-100 bpm
P Wave: Sinus   P-R Interval: Normal
QRS Complex: No axis deviation, normal voltage, no
QRS complex broadening
ST Segment: Concave ST elevation in leads V_1 to V_6
Diagnosis: Sinus rhythm, acute pericarditis

Strip 5-7   Rhythm: Regular   Rate: 60-100 bpm
P Wave: Sinus   P-R Interval: Normal
QRS Complex: No axis deviation, normal voltage, no
QRS complex broadening
ST Segment: ST segment elevation in lead aVR; ST
segment depression in many other leads

Diagnosis: Sinus rhythm, acute myocardial infarction (left coronary disease)

Strip 5-8 Rhythm: Regular   Rate: 60-100 bpm
P Wave: Sinus   P-R Interval: Normal
QRS Complex: No axis deviation, normal voltage, no QRS complex broadening
ST Segment: Convex ST elevation in leads V_1 to V_5, pathologic Q wave
Diagnosis: Sinus rhythm, acute anterior myocardial infarction

Strip 5-9 Rhythm: Regular   Rate: 60-100 bpm
P Wave: Sinus   P-R Interval: Normal
QRS Complex: No axis deviation, normal voltage, no QRS complex broadening
ST Segment: ST segment elevation in leads V_1 to V_4 (lead V_4 has returned to the baseline), pathologic Q wave
Diagnosis: Sinus rhythm, L-G-L syndrome, subacute anterior myocardial infarction

Strip 5-10 Rhythm: Regular   Rate: 60-100 bpm
P Wave: Sinus   P-R Interval: Normal
QRS Complex: No axis deviation, normal voltage, no QRS complex broadening
ST Segment: ST segment elevation in leads V_2 to V_5 (ECG abnormality found in health check of a young adult)
Diagnosis: Sinus rhythm, early repolarization syndrome

Strip 5-11   Rhythm: Regular   Rate: 60-100 bpm
P Wave: Sinus   P-R Interval: Normal
QRS Complex: No axis deviation, normal voltage, no
QRS complex broadening
ST Segment: Convex ST elevation in leads V_1 to V_5,
pathologic Q wave
Diagnosis: Sinus rhythm, acute anterior myocardial
infarction

Strip 5-12   Rhythm: Regular   Rate: 60-100 bpm
P Wave: Sinus (no related subsequent QRS complex)   P-R
Interval: Normal
QRS Complex: Right axis deviation, normal voltage,
showing M type in lead V_1, pathologic Q wave
ST Segment: Convex ST elevation in leads II, III, aVF
Diagnosis: Sinus rhythm, third degree AV block,
incomplete right bundle branch block and acute anterior
myocardial infarction

Chapter 6

T Wave

Section 1 Normal T Wave

T wave represents the rapid ventricular repolarization, also known as the ventricular recovery phase.

[ECG Recognition]

Direction:

1. T wave is usually upright in leads I, II, V_4 to V_6.

2. The morphology of T waves is variable in leads III, aVF, aVL and V_1 to V_3.

3. T wave is always inverted in lead aVR.

Amplitude:

The amplitude of T waves should not be lower than 1/10 amplitude of R wave in the same lead, except in leads III, aVL, aVF and V_1 to V_3.

[ECG Tracing: Common T Wave Waveforms] (Figure 6-1)

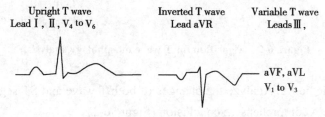

Upright T wave	Inverted T wave	Variable T wave
Lead I, II, V_4 to V_6	Lead aVR	Leads III,
		aVF, aVL
		V_1 to V_3

Figure 6-1　Normal T wave.

Above all, when analyzing T wave, the judgment should be based on the patients' history and clinical manifestation, not only the ECG, because various factors can change the morphology of T wave, and T wave change lacks specificity for diagnosis.

Section 2　Useful Methods for Analyzing T Wave

Method 1: Analyze T wave according to its morphology (peaked, flat or inverted) (Figure 6-2).

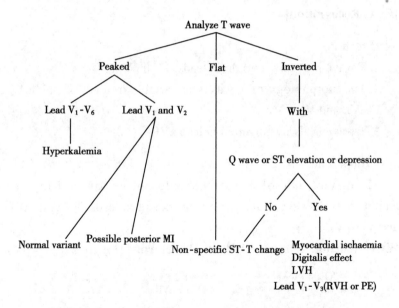

Figure 6-2　Algorithm for T wave morphology analysis.

Method 2: Analyze the changes of both T wave and ST segment to draw a comprehensive conclusion (Figure 6-3).

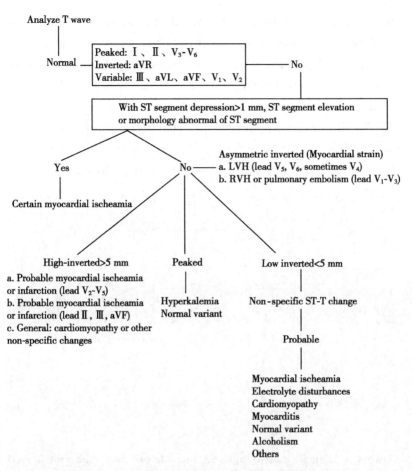

Figure 6-3　Algorithm for T wave analysis with ST segment.

Section 3　Analysis of Abnormal T Wave

Inverted T Wave

Common causes:

1. In leads Ⅰ, Ⅱ, V_4 to V_6, inverted T wave is usually abnormal.

2. If T wave is inverted with apparent change in ST segment

(horizontal or down-sloping ST segment depression >1 mm, Figure 6-3), then you can consider myocardial ischemia. Inverted T wave with ST segment depression <1 mm or down-sloping depression is non-specific, which can be caused by cardiac disease and non-cardiac disease.

　　3. Simple T wave inversion without apparent ST segment changes is non-specific under most circumstances (Figure 6-4), but the prospect for myocardial ischemia cannot be totally eliminated.

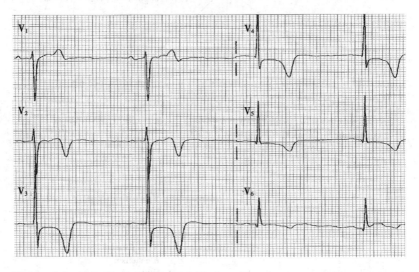

Figure 6-4　Female patient, aged 53, instable coronary syndrome onset 1 week before. Notable deep inverted T wave with convex ST segment in leads V$_2$ to V$_6$. ECG indicates myocardial infarction.

　　4. Widespread deep inverted T wave without apparent ST segment elevation or depression is not specific for diagnosis, and can be attributed to following causes: myocardial ischemia, dynamic evolution of myocardial infarction, Adams-Stroke syndrome attack, ventricular and supraventricular tachycardia attack, myocarditis, pericarditis, cardiomyopathy, pulmonary embolism, medications

(cocaine, tricyclic antidepressants,etc.), alcoholism, electrolyte disturbances, subarachnoid hemorrhage, acute pancreatitis, gallbladder disease, pheochromocytoma, etc (Figure 6-5, Figure 6-6).

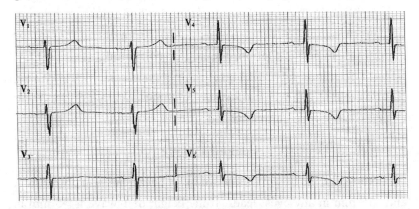

Figure 6-5   Male patient, aged 35, ECG in conventional health check. Notable inverted T wave with non-specific ST change in leads V$_4$ to V$_6$.

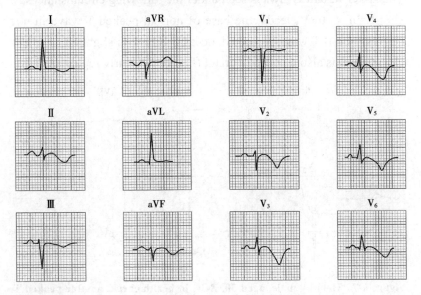

Figure 6-6   Male patient, aged 48, severe brain hemorrhage in trauma. Notable inverted T wave in most leads.

5. Symmetrical inverted T wave: the proportion of female to male is 4:1, and the common cause is myocardial ischemia, but the causes mentioned above should also be taken into consideration.

6. Slightly inverted T wave without ST segment change can be caused by the following factors, apart from above mentioned conditions: hyperventilation, feeding or cold drinks (fasting ECG is normal), mitral valve prolapse, ventricular block, pneumothorax. Besides, slight changes in T wave, without apparent ST segment changes, can still be normal variant.

Peaked T wave

Normally, the height of T wave in limb leads are usually <5 mm, and <10 mm in any chest leads. If the height of T wave is >5 mm in limb leads and >10 mm in chest leads, it is defined as peaked T wave. This ECG variant is always seen under the following circumstances:

1. In V_2 to V_5 leads, the base of normal peaked T wave in not narrow. And if T wave is peaked, occasionally with slight ST segment elevation, it is also a normal variant (Figure 6-7, early repolarization).

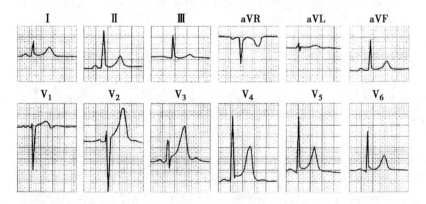

Figure 6-7   Healthy male, aged 30, ECG in health check, notable peaked T wave in leads V_2 to V_5, and prominent ST elevation in chest leads.

2. Acute myocardial ischemia or myocardial infarction (Figure 6-8, superacute phase).

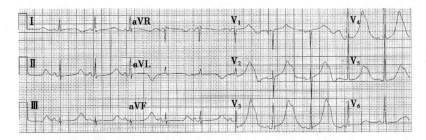

Figure 6-8   Male patient, aged 70, acute myocardial infarction, notable abnormal huge peaked T wave in chest leads.

3. Hyperkalemia (Figure 6-9).

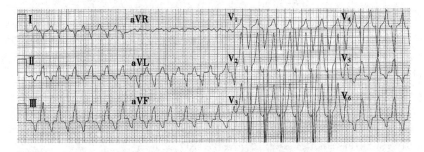

Figure 6-9   Female patient, aged 65, toxuria without regular hemodialysis, serum potassium 7.5 mmol/L during ECG examination.

4. Patients with overloaded left ventricle, such as severe mitral regurgitation.

5. Patients with cerebrovascular events (for example subarachnoid hemorrhage).

Section 4   ECG Practice Strips

Strip **6-1**   Rhythm (Regular Irregular) Rate (bpm)

P Wave (Sinus Non-sinus Absent) P-R Interval (Prolonged/Shortened)

QRS Complex (Axis Voltage Widening Absence of QRS Complex Q Wave).

ST Segment (Elevated/Depressed) T wave (Peaked/Flat/Lower)

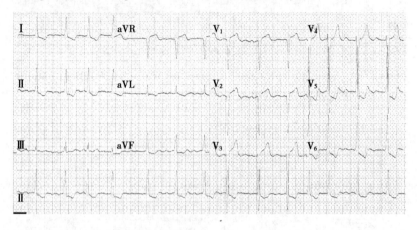

Strip **6-2**   Rhythm (Regular Irregular) Rate (bpm)

P Wave (Sinus Non-sinus Absent) P-R Interval (Prolonged/Shortened)

QRS Complex (Axis Voltage Widening Absence of QRS Complex Q Wave)

ST Segment (Elevated/Depressed) T wave (Peaked/Flat/Lower)

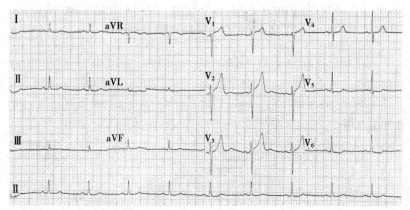

Strip **6-3**   Rhythm (Regular   Irregular)   Rate (bpm)

P Wave (Sinus   Non-sinus   Absent)   P-R Interval (Prolonged/Shortened)

QRS Complex (Axis   Voltage   Widening   Absence of QRS Complex   Q Wave)

ST Segment (Elevated/Depressed)   T wave (Peaked/Flat/Flattened)

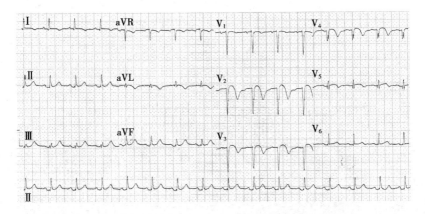

Strip **6-4**   Rhythm (Regular   Irregular)   Rate (bpm)

P Wave (Sinus   Non-sinus   Absent)   P-R Interval (Prolonged/Shortened)

QRS Complex (Axis   Voltage   Widening   Absence of QRS Complex   Q Wave)

ST Segment (Elevated/Depressed)   T wave (Peaked/Flat/Flattened)

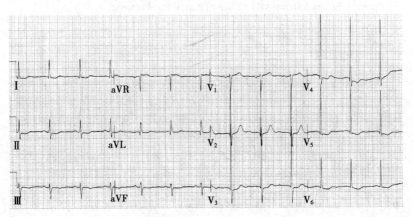

Strip **6-5** Rhythm (Regular Irregular) Rate (bpm)
P Wave (Sinus Non-sinus Absent) P-R Interval (Prolonged/Shortened)
QRS Complex (Axis Voltage Widening Absence of QRS Complex Q Wave)
ST Segment (Elevated/Depressed) T wave (Peaked/Flat/Flattened)

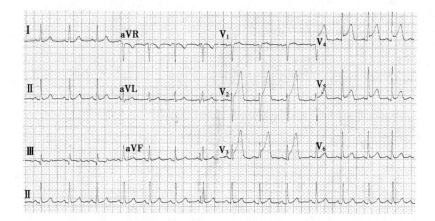

Strip **6-6** Rhythm (Regular Irregular) Rate (bpm)
P Wave (Sinus Non-sinus Absent) P-R Interval (Prolonged/Shortened)
QRS Complex (Axis Voltage Widening Absence of QRS Complex Q Wave)
ST Segment (Elevated/Depressed) T wave (Peaked/Flat/Flattened)

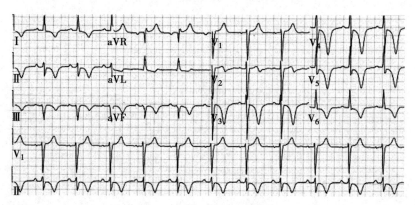

Strip **6-7**　Rhythm (Regular　Irregular)　Rate (　　bpm)
P Wave (Sinus　Non-sinus　Absent)　P-R Interval (Prolonged/Shortened)
QRS Complex (Axis　Voltage　Widening　Absence of QRS Complex　Q Wave)
ST Segment (Elevated/Depressed)　T wave (Peaked/Flat/Flattened)

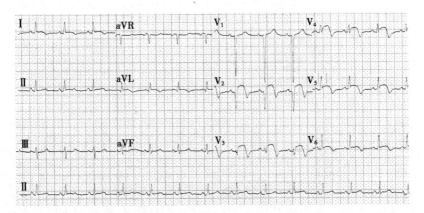

Strip **6-8**　Rhythm (Regular　Irregular)　Rate (　　bpm)
P Wave (Sinus　Non-sinus　Absent)　P-R Interval (Prolonged/Shortened)
QRS Complex (Axis　Voltage　Widening　Absence of QRS Complex　Q Wave)
ST Segment (Elevated/Depressed)　T wave (Peaked/Flat/Flattened)

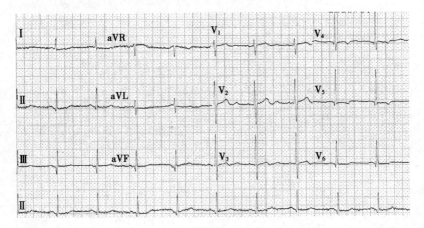

Strip **6-9** Rhythm (Regular Irregular) Rate (bpm)
P Wave (Sinus Non-sinus Absent) P-R Interval (Prolonged/Shortened)
QRS Complex (Axis Voltage Widening Absence of QRS Complex Q Wave)
ST Segment (Elevated/Depressed) T wave (Peaked/Flat/Flattened)

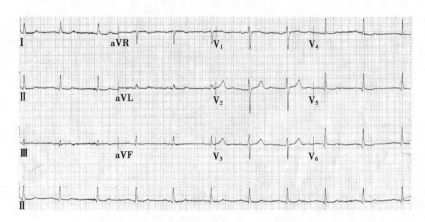

Strip **6-10** Rhythm (Regular Irregular) Rate (bpm)
P Wave (Sinus Non-sinus Absent) P-R Interval (Prolonged/Shortened)
QRS Complex (Axis Voltage Widening Absence of QRS Complex Q Wave)
ST Segment (Elevated/Depressed) T wave (Peaked/Flat/Flattened)

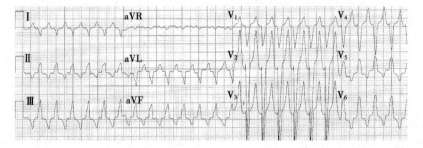

Answers to the Strips

Strip 6-1   Rhythm: Regular   Rate: More than 100 bpm

P Waves: Not sinus   P-R Interval: Normal

QRS Complex: No axis deviation, abnormal voltage ($R_{V5}+S_{V1}>4.0$ mV), no notable widening)

ST Segment:'Hook'ST

T wave: Inverted T waves in leads I , II , aVL, aVF, V_5 to V_6

Diagnosis: Atrial fibrillation, left ventricular hypertrophy, digitalis effect, T wave change (caused by ventricular hypertrophy, a sign of myocardial strain)

Strip 6-2   Rhythm: Regular   Rate: 60 to 100 bpm

P Waves: Sinus   P-R Interval: Normal

QRS Complex: No axis deviation, normal voltage in all leads, no notable widening)

ST Segment: Normal

T wave: Peaked T waves in leads V_1 to V_3

Diagnosis: Sinus rhythm, normal ECG

Strip 6-3   Rhythm: Regular   Rate: 60 to 100 bpm

P Waves: Sinus   P-R Interval: Normal

QRS Complex: No axis deviation, normal voltage in all leads, no notable widening)

ST Segment: Convex ST segment elevation in leads V_1 to V_5, pathologic Q wave appears

T wave: Inverted T waves in leads V_1 to V_5

Diagnosis: Sinus rhythm, acute anterior myocardium infarction

Strip 6-4　Rhythm: Regular　Rate: 60 to 100 bpm
P Waves: Sinus　P-R Interval: Normal
QRS Complex: No axis deviation, normal voltage in all
leads, no notable widening)
ST Segment: Depression in leads V_3 to V_6
T wave: Inverted T waves in leads V_4 to V_6
Diagnosis: Sinus rhythm, left ventricular hypertrophy, T wave
change (caused by ventricular hypertrophy, a sign of strain)

Strip 6-5　Rhythm: Regular　Rate: 60 to 100 bpm
P Waves: Sinus　P-R Interval: Normal
QRS Complex: No axis deviation, normal voltage in all
leads, no notable widening)
ST Segment: Concave ST segment elevation in leads V_1 to V_6
T wave: Peaked T waves in leads V_1 to V_6
Diagnosis: Sinus rhythm, acute pericarditis

Strip 6-6　Rhythm: Regular　Rate: 60 to 100 bpm
P Waves: Sinus　P-R Interval: Normal
QRS Complex: No axis deviation, normal voltage in all
leads, no notable widening)
ST Segment: Slight elevation in leads V_2 to V_5
T wave: Widespread inverted T wave in leads V_2 to V_5
Diagnosis: Sinus rhythm, subarachnoid hemorrhage

Strip 6-7　Rhythm: Regular　Rate: 60 to 100 bpm
P Waves: Sinus　P-R Interval: Normal
QRS Complex: No axis deviation, normal voltage in all
leads, no notable widening)
ST Segment: Convex ST segment elevation in leads V_1 to

V_5, pathologic Q wave appears

T wave: Widespread inverted T wave in leads V_2 to V_5

Diagnosis: Sinus rhythm, acute anterior myocardium infarction

Strip 6-8   Rhythm: Regular   Rate: 60 to 100 bpm

P Waves: Sinus   P-R Interval: Normal

QRS Complex: No axis deviation, normal voltage in all leads, no notable widening)

ST Segment: Normal

T wave: Inverted T wave in leads V_4 to V_6

Diagnosis: Sinus rhythm, normal ECG (non-specific T wave change)

Strip 6-9   Rhythm: Regular   Rate: 60 to 100 bpm

P Waves: Sinus   P-R Interval: Normal

QRS Complex: No axis deviation, normal voltage in all leads, no notable widening)

ST Segment: Normal

T wave: Flattened T waves in leads V_4 to V_6

Diagnosis: Sinus rhythm, normal ECG (non-specific T wave change)

Strip 6-10   Rhythm: Regular   Rate: More than 100 bpm

P Waves: Absent

QRS Complex: Axis right deviation, normal voltage in all leads, notable widening)

ST Segment: Normal

T wave: Peaked T waves in leads V_1 to V_6

Diagnosis: Sinus rhythm, hyperkalemia

Chapter 7

Other Common Abnormal ECGs

Section 1   Q-T Interval

Q-T interval represents the total time from ventricular depolarization to repolarization. The prolongation of Q-T interval indicates the prolongation of ventricular repolarization, and reentrant arrhythmia, for example torsade de pointes, is likely to take place during this interval.

Common causes of Q-T interval prolongation:

- Congenital long Q-T interval syndrome.
- Acquired long Q-T interval syndrome.

Non-drug-related reasons: Myocardial ischemia, central nervous system disorders, severe bradyarrhythmia, hypokalemia.

Drug-related reasons: Type I a, I c and III antiarrhythmia medications, erythromycin, non- sedative antihistamines (e.g. astemizole and terfenadine).

Common causes of Q-T interval shortening (lacks of clinical evidence):

1. Digitalis overdose.
2. Hypercalcemia.
3. Short Q-T interval syndrome.

[ECG Recognition]

1. Q-T interval is affected by heart rate. Q-Tc needs to be calculated, which represents the actual Q-T interval when

the rate is 60 bpm. Q-Tc=Q-T/√R-R.

2. The normal heart rate is between 60 and 100 bpm, and normal Q-T interval is between 0.32 and 0.44s.

[ECG Tracing] (Figure 7-1)

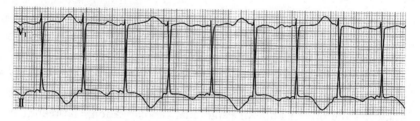

Figure 7-1   Prolonged Q-T interval.

Section 2   Hyperkalemia

[ECG Recognition]

1. Mild Hyperkalemia: when the serum potassium level is approximately between 5.7 and 6.5 mmol/L, P wave widens; tall, peaked, narrow-base and tented T waves occur in many leads; P-R interval prolongs, and first-degree AVB can happen.

2. Severe Hyperkalemia: when serum potassium level is over 6.5 mmol/L, the latter portion of the QRS complex is significantly widened, which shows marked notching or slurring. As a result, the widened QRS will merge with tall and tented T wave, and ST segment will be elevated.

3. High-degree AVB: P wave disappears.

4. Ventricular tachycardia, ventricular fibrillation or autonomous ventricular rhythm.

[ECG Tracing] (Figure 7-2)

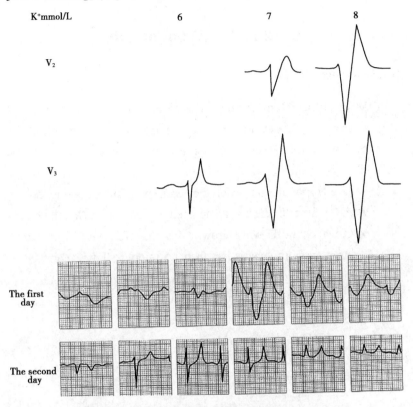

Figure 7-2　Different levels of hyperkalemia.

Day 1, the serum potassium level is 8.6 mmol/L: P wave disappeared, and QRS complex broadened obviously. Day 2, the serum potassium level is 5.8 mmol/L: P wave is present; P-R interval lengthened; QRS complex is normal and T wave is tented.

　　1. Serum potassium>6.0 mmol/L: the earliest change is that T wave tends to be tall, narrow-based and tented, and P-R interval may be prolonged.

　　2. Serum potassium>7.0 mmol/L: P wave flattens or disappears; QRS complex widens; and prominent S wave can be seen.

　　3. Serum potassium>8.0 mmol/L: S wave widens and deepens

progressively, and the ST segment is steeper; no ST segment is isoelectric.

Section 3　Hypokalemia

[ECG Recognition]

1. Mild Hypokalemia: when the serum potassium level is approximately between 3.0 and 3.5 mmol/L, the amplitude of T wave decreases progressively, and the amplitude of U wave is as small as T wave.

2. Severe Hypokalemia: when the serum potassium level is less than 3.0 mmol/L, there is an apparent increase in the amplitude of U wave, and U wave grows taller than T wave. When the serum potassium level is less than 1.5 mmol/L, T wave and U wave can merge, which is most obvious in leads V_2 to V_5.

3. ST segment depresses progressively.

4. QRS complex duration is prolonged.

5. P-R interval is slightly prolonged.

[ECG Tracing] (Figure 7-3)

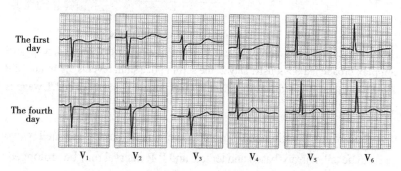

Figure 7-3　Different levels of hypokalemia.

Day 1, serum potassium level is 1.5 mmol/L: T wave and U wave are fused; U wave is obvious and QU interval prolongs. Day 2, serum potassium level is 3.7 mmol/L: the ECG returned to be normal.

Section 4   Digitalis Effect

Digitalis is an effective medication used in treating heart failure and some arrhythmias. Digitalis effect refers to the shortening of Q-T interval and ST-T changes in ECG after taking therapeutic dosage (Figure 7-4).

[ECG Recognition]

1. ST segment depresses, which is concave upward, hook-like change.
2. T wave can be biphasic with its amplitude decrease.
3. The Q-T interval is shortened.
4. The P-R interval prolongs: first-degree AVB.
5. U wave increases in height.

[ECG Tracing] (Figure 7-4)

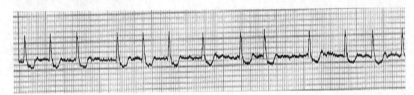

Figure 7-4   Digitalis effect ECG.

Section 5   Electrical Alternans

Electrical alternans refers to the ECG variant on which consecutive QRS complexes alternate in the amplitude, direction or pattern in any lead or all leads, while the R-R interval remains unchanged. Some common causes of electrical alternans are shown below:

1. The electrical alternans of QRS complex is relatively rare in patients with cardiac tamponade, but it can be seen in patients with large amount of pericardial effusions, especially in some patients with malignant tumors.

2. Complete electrical alternans is highly suggestive of cardiac tamponade, but it only occur in fewer than 10% of cardiac tamponade cases.

3. Severe coronary artery disease (CAD) and hypertrophic cardiomyopathy (HCM) are uncommon causes for alternans.

4. Electrical alternans is also associated with supraventricular tachycardia (SVT) with fast ventricular rate (usually can be seen in WPW syndrome orthodromic AVRT).

[ECG Recognition]

1. Consecutive QRS complexes alternate in the amplitude, direction or pattern in any lead or all leads, while the R-R interval remains unchanged.

2. If electrical alternans occurs on all P waves, QRS complex and T waves (sometimes including U waves), it is defined as complete electrical alternans.

[ECG Tracing] (Figure 7-5)

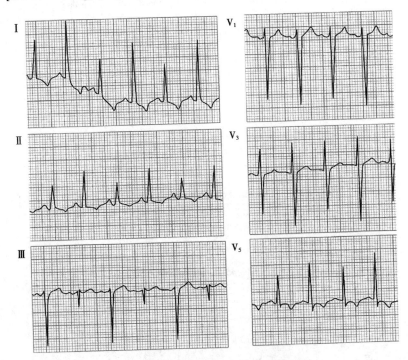

Figure 7-5   Electrical alternans ECG.

Section 6   ECG Practice Strips

Strip **7-1**   Rhythm (Regular   Irregular)   Rate (bpm)

P Wave (Sinus   Non-sinus   Absent)   P-R Interval (Prolonged/Shortened)

QRS Complex (Axis   Voltage   Widening   Absence of QRS Complex   Q Wave)

ST Segment (Elevated/Depressed)

T wave (Peaked/Flat/Flattened)

Other abnormalities (Q-T interval/Hypokalemia/Hyperkalemia)

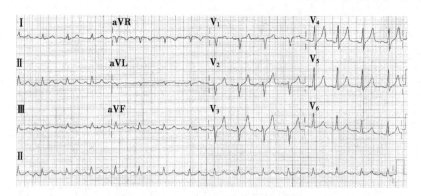

Strip 7-2   Rhythm (Regular   Irregular)   Rate (bpm)

P Wave (Sinus   Non-sinus   Absent)   P-R Interval (Prolonged/Shortened)

QRS Complex (Axis   Voltage   Widening   Absence of QRS Complex   Q Wave)

ST Segment (Elevated/Depressed)

T wave (Peaked/Flat/Flattened)

Other abnormalities (Q-T interval/Hypokalemia/Hyperkalemia)

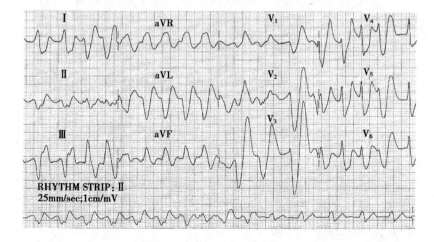

Strip **7-3**   Rhythm (Regular   Irregular)   Rate (bpm)

P Wave (Sinus   Non-sinus   Absent)   P-R Interval (Prolonged/Shortened)

QRS Complex (Axis   Voltage   Widening   Absence of QRS Complex   Q Wave)

ST Segment (Elevated/Depressed)

T wave (Peaked/Flat/Flattened)

Other abnormalities (Q-T interval/Hypokalemia/Hyperkalemia)

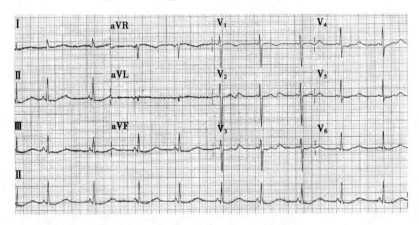

Strip **7-4**   Rhythm (Regular   Irregular)   Rate (bpm)

P Wave (Sinus   Non-sinus   Absent)   P-R Interval (Prolonged/Shortened)

QRS Complex (Axis   Voltage   Widening   Absence of QRS Complex   Q Wave)

ST Segment (Elevated/Depressed)

T wave (Peaked/Flat/Flattened)

Other abnormalities (Q-T interval/Hypokalemia/Hyperkalemia)

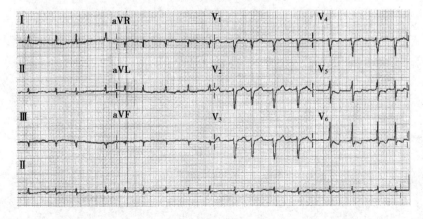

Strip **7-5** Rhythm (Regular Irregular) Rate (bpm)

P Wave (Sinus Non-sinus Absent) P-R Interval (Prolonged/Shortened)

QRS Complex (Axis Voltage Widening Absence of QRS Complex Q Wave)

ST Segment (Elevated/Depressed)

T wave (Peaked/Flat/Flattened)

Other abnormalities (Q-T interval/Hypokalemia/Hyperkalemia)

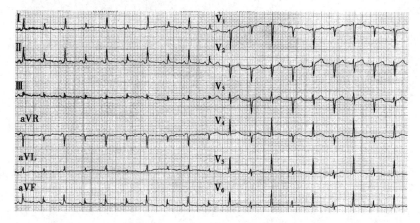

Strip **7-6** Rhythm (Regular Irregular) Rate (bpm)

P Wave (Sinus Non-sinus Absent) P-R Interval (Prolonged/Shortened)

QRS Complex (Axis Voltage Widening Absence of QRS Complex Q Wave)

ST Segment (Elevated/Depressed)

T wave (Peaked/Flat/Flattened)

Other abnormalities (Q-T interval/Hypokalemia/Hyperkalemia)

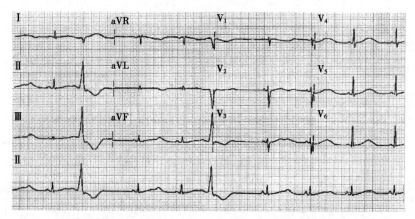

Answers to the Strips

Strip 7-1   Rhythm: Regular   Rate: 60 to 100 bpm
P Waves: Sinus   P-R Interval: Normal
QRS Complex: No axis deviation, abnormal voltage in
chest leads, no notable widening
ST Segment: Normal
T wave: Peaked T waves in leads V_1 to V_6
Diagnosis: Sinus rhythm, hyperkalemia

Strip 7-2   Rhythm: Regular   Rate: More than 100 bpm
P Waves: Not sinus
QRS Complex: No axis deviation, abnormal voltage in
chest leads, notable widening
ST Segment: Normal
T wave: Peaked T waves in most leads
Diagnosis: Sinus tachycardia, hyperkalemia

Strip 7-3   Rhythm: Regular   Rate: 60 to 100 bpm
P Waves: Sinus   P-R Interval: Normal
QRS Complex: No axis deviation, abnormal voltage in
chest leads, no notable widening
ST Segment: Normal
T wave: Normal
Other abnormalities: U waves in leads V_1 to V_6
Diagnosis: Sinus rhythm, hypokalemia

Strip 7-4   Rhythm: Irregular   Rate: 60 to 100 bpm
P Waves: Sinus   P-R Interval: Normal
QRS Complex: No axis deviation, abnormal voltage in

chest leads, no notable widening

ST Segment: Oblique depression in leads V_4 to V_6, "hook" ST

T wave: Inversion in leads V_4 to V_6

Diagnosis: Atrial fibrillation, digitalis effect

Strip 7-5   Rhythm: Regular   Rate: More than 100 bpm

P Waves: Not sinus   P-R interval: Normal

QRS Complex: No axis deviation, abnormal voltage in all leads, no notable widening

ST Segment: Normal

T wave: Normal

Diagnosis: Sinus tachycardia, electrical alternans

Strip 7-6   Rhythm: Regular   Rate: 60 to 100 bpm

P Waves: Sinus   P-R Interval: Normal

QRS Complex: No axis deviation, normal voltage in all leads, notable widening and appears in advance

ST Segment: Normal

T wave: Normal

Other abnormalities: Q-T interval is prolonged obviously

Diagnosis: Sinus rhythm, premature ventricular contraction, long Q-T syndrome